*Enhancing Human Traits*

# Hastings Center Studies in Ethics

## A SERIES EDITED BY

# Mark J. Hanson and Daniel Callahan

This series of books, published by The Hastings Center and Georgetown University Press, examines ethical issues in medicine and the life sciences. Established in 1969, The Hastings Center, located in Garrison, New York, is an independent, nonprofit, and nonpartisan research organization. The work of the Center is mainly carried out through research projects, the publication of the *Hastings Center Report* and *IRB: A Review of Human Subjects Research*, and numerous workshops, conferences, lectures, and consultations. **The Hastings Center Studies in Ethics** series brings the ongoing research of The Hastings Center to a wider audience.

# Enhancing Human Traits:

## Ethical and Social Implications

EDITED BY
Erik Parens

GEORGETOWN UNIVERSITY PRESS / WASHINGTON, D.C.

Georgetown University Press, Washington, D.C. 20007
© 1998 by Georgetown University Press. All rights reserved.
Printed in the United States of America
10   9   8   7   6   5   4   3   2   1                    1998
THIS VOLUME IS PRINTED ON ACID FREE ⊗ OFFSET BOOK PAPER

**Library of Congress Cataloging-in-Publication Data**

Enhancing human traits : ethical and social implications / edited by
    Erik Parens.
        p.    cm.—(Hastings Center studies in ethics)
    Includes bibliographical references.
    ISBN 0-87840-703-0
    1. Medical innovations—Moral and ethical aspects.  2. Medical
innovations—Social aspects.  3. Psychotropic drugs—Moral and
ethical aspects.  4. Surgery, Plastic—Moral and ethical aspects.
5. Performance technology—Moral and ethical aspects.    I. Parens,
Erik, 1957–   .    II. Series.
RA418.5.M4E54    1998
174'.25—dc21                                             98-16197

# CONTENTS

# *Introduction*

At a Hastings Center meeting in 1993, LeRoy Walters gave a presentation on "enhancement." He invited his audience to suspend disbelief and imagine four scenarios. The first, which involved a genetic intervention that could "enhance" our ability to resist disease, inspired little controversy. If one can assume that all persons will have equal access to such a new form of prevention, then it's difficult to see what the worries might be.

About the second scenario, however, there was some controversy. Here Walters invited us to imagine a genetic intervention that could "enhance" our ability to be alert without needing to sleep as much as we do now. Anybody with young children can appreciate how terrific it might be to need less sleep. But wouldn't sleeping less mean dreaming less? Would that be a good thing? And what sorts of projects would we expect ourselves to pursue with the extra time?

The third scenario also raised some concern. Here Walters invited us to imagine a genetic intervention that could "enhance" our long-term memory. Anyone past thirty-five can appreciate the benefits of that intervention. But would such an enhancement also mean that one would be saddled forever with some memories one would rather forget?

None of the scenarios raised controversy like the last. Here Walters asked us to suppose that there was a genetic intervention "aimed at reducing the ferocious tendencies of human beings and increasing their generous tendencies." Such an intervention could compensate for "a tragic, perhaps even fatal, evolutionary flaw in our species." At this point at least one member of the audience nearly blew a gasket. You mean you think we're wise enough to know what level of generosity we ought to try to achieve with a new genetic technology? Mightn't a genetic intervention aimed at enhancing generosity inadvertently eliminate, say, the capacity for creativity or the desire for distinction? Are we so confident in the wisdom of our conceptions of normality and perfection that we are prepared to use new genetic technologies to achieve them?

Several months after Walters's talk at The Hastings Center, Peter Kramer's book *Listening to Prozac* shot to the top of the *New York Times* best seller list. That book thoughtfully explored some of the reasons why one might worry about a drug that can make some individuals feel not just well, but "better than well." In the end, Kramer rather enthusiastically exhorted his readers to accept that since we *can* now "enhance" ourselves with new biotechnologies like Prozac, it is time to start thinking about how we *should* enhance ourselves.

And Kramer's advice is reasonable. There is no good reason to think that we'll decide altogether to stop using the biotechnological means we've already got, or that we won't invest in the creation of new ones. Moreover, no matter how many worries one might have about some of the "enhancement" purposes to which the new biotechnological means are and will be put, one has to remember that, in general and by definition, enhancement is the sort of thing we endorse.

Thus late 1993 seemed like a good time to try to ask a very basic question about aiming new biotechnologies at enhancement purposes: Given that much of human history can be seen as the pursuit of one or another kind of "enhancement," and given that much of that history is strewn with needless worry about putatively "dangerous" new technologies, will there ever be good reasons to worry about new biotechnologies aimed at the enhancement of human capacities? To begin to grapple with that question, in 1995 The Hastings Center received a grant from the National Endowment for the Humanities (RH-21271-95) to do a project, "On the Prospect of Technologies Aimed at the Enhancement of Human Capacities." One of the major outcomes of that project is the present volume. Its purpose is to enable you, too, to begin to grapple with the conceptual and ethical issues that surround the prospect of aiming new biotechnologies at the enhancement of human capacities and traits.

In addition to ongoing research by and conversation among the project participants, our two-year project entailed four major research meetings. At those meetings, papers were presented and discussed at length. Revised versions of most of those papers appear in this volume. In keeping with the customary method of The Hastings Center, the papers are written from different disciplines. As is inevitably the case when one brings together people who are not only from different disciplines but who have different perspectives and commitments, there were substantive disagreements. For an account of some of these disagreements please see my essay *Is Better Always Good? The Enhancement*

*Project.* This paper (which was previously published as a special supplement to the *Hastings Center Report* 28, no. 1 [1998]) gives an overview of the work of the project as well as my own tentative conclusions based on that work.

The remaining essays in this volume constitute the major papers presented at the meetings. The first two are devoted to the uses and meanings of the term *enhancement.* Anyone who has attempted to engage in a conversation about enhancement knows how slippery the term can be. Eric Juengst provides a very helpful account of how it means different things in different interpretive and social contexts. Dan Brock elucidates the sorts of conceptual and practical complexities that policymakers will have to bear in mind when they employ the term.

The next three essays explore the dangers that attend any attempt to employ the term *enhancement* in policy contexts. David Frankford investigates his concern that the term, as part of the treatment/enhancement distinction, will be used by insurers to refuse people services they need—as in, "you don't need that service, it's just an enhancement." In her interrogation of Norman Daniels's work, Anita Silvers explores her concern that embedded in the notion of enhancement is a deeply problematic valorization of "the normal." Kathy Davis describes the difficulties that policymakers in The Netherlands encountered when they attempted to use the treatment/enhancement distinction to help articulate what should be considered part of a basic package of care.

The ethical implications in the policy debate raise another question that is often present, but not explicitly explored, in conversations about enhancement, namely: Is there anything morally new or significant about new biotechnological means? Can it ever make sense to worry about putting new biotechnological means to what look like ancient and morally acceptable ends? If, for example, an ancient end of schools has been to enhance student learning, what could be problematic about a new pharmacological agent that helped to achieve that ancient end? Carol Freedman takes up the particular question regarding the new psychopharmacological means Prozac, and investigates how it is similar to and different from traditional means like psychotherapy. In more general terms, Ronald Cole-Turner explores the moral difference that new biotechnological means might make.

Assuming that there are no "uniquely" new ethical or social problems, the next two essays explore some of the familiar ethical and social problems that new biotechnologies can exacerbate. Carl Elliott explores how psychopharmacological agents like Prozac can be used to promote

fairly particular conceptions of a good life. Margaret Olivia Little investigates how cosmetic surgery can make purchasers and practitioners
become complicit with what she calls "suspect" conceptions of normality,
while from a vastly different perspective and in a very different mode,
Susan Bordo articulates the same concern in "*Braveheart, Babe,* and the
Body: Contemporary Images of the Body." Bordo presented an early
version of that essay at our second project meeting; she then published
it her book, *Twilight Zone: The Hidden Life of Cultural Images from Plato
to O.J.* (Berkeley: University of California Press, 1997). We reprint
that essay here with permission of the author and the University of
California Press.

The volume's final papers broach the daunting question, What sort
of people do we want to become? Gerald McKenny reviews some of
the dominant Western philosophical conceptions of how medicine should
use technology to respond to the vulnerability of human bodies. In so
doing he shows the often underappreciated ethical significance of those
responses. Like McKenny, Mary Winkler also undertakes her exploration in a rich historical context. While Winkler has concerns (as does
McKenny) about using biotechnologies to enhance our capacities and
traits, she does not argue for the blanket prohibition of any given
enhancement purpose. Rather, like the project as a whole, she tries to
articulate as clearly as possible what is ethically at stake when we use
new biotechnologies to achieve such purposes. She helps us ask the
right questions.

If it weren't for LeRoy Walters's talk on enhancement in 1993 at
The Hastings Center, the energy necessary to drive thinking about a
project might not have been generated. If it weren't for Daniel Callahan's
guidance and nudging, the grant application to the NEH would not
have been finished. And if it weren't for the careful administrative work
of Nicole Rozanski, this volume would not have made it to John
Samples's office at the Georgetown University Press. I am indebted to
those individuals, to the contributors to this volume, and to the following
individuals who also made presentations and/or attended project meetings: W. French Anderson, Adrienne Asch, Erika Blacksher, Bette
Crigger, Eve DeVaro, Lawrence Diller, Strachan Donnelley, Harold
Edgar, Mark Hanson, Bruce Jennings, Peter Kramer, Sheldon Krimsky,
Tracy Macdonald, Glen McGee, Ellen Moskowitz, Leigh Turner, Lawrence Vogel, LeRoy Walters, and Peter Whitehouse.

ERIK PARENS

ERIK PARENS

# Is Better Always Good?
# The Enhancement Project

Worry about enhancement? Why not worry instead about apple pie? Enhancement, after all, is something we seek for ourselves and think others should too. We praise individuals who exercise so that they will live longer, be thinner, and if not richer, at least happier. We applaud individuals who seek excellent schools to enhance their intellectual development. We praise parents who do everything they can to enhance their children's moral development. So why would anyone worry about a new cosmetic surgery technique that promised to make us thinner? Why worry about a new psychopharmacological agent that promised to enhance concentration and performance in school? What about a new psychopharmacological or genetic technology that promised to make us kinder and gentler?[1]

The following essay begins to say why and when it will sometimes make sense to worry about the prospect of aiming new biotechnologies at the enhancement of human capacities and traits. When we began our two-year project funded by the National Endowment for the Humanities,[2] we hoped to articulate for policymakers what we called "a continuum of uses of 'enhancement technologies,' from those that promote shared values, to those that seem neither to promote nor threaten shared values, to those that threaten such values." That hope was misguided in a couple of ways. First, it failed to appreciate that the heterogeneity of the technologies and the number of problems surrounding their regulation make the idea of "a continuum" unrealistic. Second, the phrase "enhancement technologies" itself is potentially misleading. The phrase could be read to suggest that "enhancement technologies" are in a class different from, say, the class of "health technologies." But of course they are not. The same technology can be aimed at different purposes. A genetic technology that could increase muscle mass for the purpose of treating a patient with a degenerative muscle disease could also be used to enhance the ability of an athlete to compete at lifting weights.

In a word, we quickly discovered that our project's primary aim should be to help clear some of the conceptual ground. This purpose entailed not only trying to clarify the different ways in which the term *enhancement* is used, but trying to clarify some good reasons why anyone might worry about aiming new biotechnologies at the enhancement of human capacities and traits.

One of the things we learned is that to understand worries about enhancement, one needs to notice that the term *enhancement* is used in at least two different, albeit sometimes overlapping, sorts of conversations—and for different reasons. In the first sort of conversation, enhancement is one pole of the treatment/enhancement distinction. It is used in conversations by people attempting to say what doctors, as doctors, should and shouldn't do or by people attempting to say what a just system of health insurance should and shouldn't provide. This conversation is often conducted, explicitly or implicitly, in terms of the proper goals of medicine.

In the second sort of conversation the concern is not primarily that doctors might provide an intervention that would undermine the proper goals of the profession. Rather, the concern is that anyone who provided the intervention would be undermining extramedical, social goals or would be exacerbating already existing social problems. The first half of this essay is devoted to enhancement as it appears in conversations about the goals of medicine; the second half is devoted to enhancement as it appears in conversations about what might be called the goals of society.

In the essay that follows I draw heavily on the work of the project participants, but do not claim that all would share my conclusions. In particular, some participants think the term *enhancement* is so freighted with erroneous assumptions and so ripe for abuse that we ought not even to use it. My sense is that if we didn't use enhancement, we would end up with another term with similar problems. Rather than attempt to come up with a term that is free of such problems, it is my view that we ought to begin with what we've got, and try to articulate as clearly as possible what the dangerous and problematic uses are. I elaborate such uses below, but invite the reader to consult the essays that follow. Indeed nearly every aspect of my overview is elaborated in at least one of these essays.

## Enhancement and the Goals of Medicine

As mentioned above, the treatment/enhancement distinction is often used in the context of conversations about what falls within and what falls outside the proper goals of medicine. But as anyone who has participated in or observed such a conversation knows, there is no one universally accepted conception of the goals of medicine. The lack of such a consensus has much to do with the fact that there is no one universally accepted conception of what health is. And thus neither is there a universally accepted definition of what "going beyond health to enhancement" means.

Within the goals of medicine conversation, there is, in the starkest terms, a long-standing debate between those who view health as freedom from disease and those who, like the authors of the famous World Health Organization definition, view health as "a state of complete physical, mental, and social well-being." In Norman Daniels and James Sabin's terms, there is a long-standing debate between "hard-line" and "expansive" conceptions of health, and thus between "hard-line" and "expansive" conceptions of the goals of medicine in particular and of health care more generally.[3]

### The Treatment/Enhancement Distinction and the Normal Function Model

Perhaps the most persuasive defender of the "hard-line"—or "normal function"—view is Norman Daniels. On this view, "disease and disability are seen as departures from species-typical normal functional organization or functioning."[4] As Daniels puts it, "According to the normal function model, the central purpose of health care is to maintain, restore, or compensate for the restricted opportunity and loss of function caused by disease and disability. Successful health care restores people to the range of opportunities they would have had without the pathological condition or prevents further deterioration."[5] One of the roots of this view is the conviction that the primary aim of health care is to provide people with normal function so that they can have an "equal opportunity" to pursue their life plans.

The terms "normal" and "equal" can be a bit confusing here. At the heart of the normal function model is the view that health care ought to help people become "normal"—which is not to say "equal"—competitors. Crudely put, the normal function model accepts that people are unequally endowed with respect to traits and talents; it accepts that "by nature" individuals are not equal competitors. The normal function model insists, rather, that those unequal competitors are entitled to an equal opportunity to pursue their life plans within the limits set by those natural endowments. On this view, medicine's primary goal is to restore people to the normal function that disease and disability diminish and which is the necessary condition for them to pursue their life plans.

Proceeding from such a conception of health, disease, and the goals of medicine (and health care), Daniels writes: "Characterizing medical need [as what has to be done to restore species-typical functioning] implies a contrast between medical services that *treat* disease (or disability) conditions and uses that merely *enhance* human performance or appearance"[6] (emphasis added).

There are at least two uses of the distinction between interventions that aim at treatment and interventions that aim at enhancement, between interventions that aim at the restoration of species-typical function and enhancements that aim at something more. The primary use, and the one that motivates Daniels, is as a tool to articulate what just health care entails. On his account, a just and basic package of care would include treatments but exclude enhancements. A just system of national health care insurance, for example, would cover the former but not the latter.

The second use is as a tool in the fight against medicalization. That is, the normal function model helps to identify the proper domain of medicine—such that some forms of disease are beyond its proper reach. Daniels and Sabin introduce an example of what I mean in their essay, "Determining 'Medical Necessity' in Mental Health Practice."[7] They point out that many different kinds of shyness can produce dis-ease in this society. The normal function conception enables us to distinguish among such kinds: to distinguish, for example, between shyness that is caused by "illness" and hence deserves treatment, and shyness that is caused by "life" and which, while worthy of response, does not deserve the services of a health care system with limited resources. As Daniels and Sabin point out, in contrast to expansive models of the goals of medicine, the normal function model enables us to make a "moral distinction between [the] treatment of illness and [the] enhancement of disadvantageous personal capabilities" (p. 10).

According to the normal function model, "complete physical, mental, and social well-being" is beyond the proper domain of medicine. The ability to identify what is beyond medicine's proper domain is enormously appealing to people who worry that too much is being brought within it. Insofar as the normal function model accepts that people are thrown into the world with different endowments, it can be a tool to fight medicalization; it can help us to remember that there are natural differences and characteristics that medicine ought not to be used to erase.

### Problems with the Treatment/Enhancement Distinction

As do all distinctions and models, however, this version[8] of the treatment/enhancement distinction and the normal function model has several problems—having to do with the intelligibility of the distinction and with the assumptions embedded in it, as well as with the uses to which it might be put by unreflective policymakers.

One of the first problems with Daniels's version of the treatment/ enhancement distinction is that it can be confusing: both interventions aimed at treating disease and ones aimed at enhancing human performance are *improvements*. That may be one reason why LeRoy Walters and Julie Palmer have chosen, instead of distinguishing between treatments and enhancements, to distinguish between health-related enhancements and nonhealth-related enhancements.[9] There are at least a couple of virtues to this approach. First, Walters and Palmer's distinction conveys the sense that both sorts of intervention are improvements over an existing condition: one is health related and the other isn't. Second, the category of health-related enhancement is large enough to accommodate treatment and prevention—a virtue for those who worry that "enhancements" aimed at preventing disease (such as vaccines) will be pointed to as a way to undermine altogether the notion that enhancement is a class worthy of special attention. The downside is that the new version of the treatment/enhancement distinction may obscure the fact that the health-related enhancement/nonhealth-related enhancement distinction carries very similar difficulties (for example, what is the difference between health- and nonhealth-related traits?) and thus just postpones having to deal with them. While our group did not reach any consensus about this matter, it may be that rather than try to craft a single term such as health-related enhancement to encompass treatment and prevention, we should just concede that we need to add to the categories treatment (of disease) and enhancement a third: prevention (of disease).[10]

A second, widely discussed problem with Daniels's account of the treatment/enhancement distinction is that it can appear to be arbitrary.

To make that point, David B. Allen and Norm Fost offer the follow-ing scenario:

> Johnny is a short eleven-year-old boy with documented growth-hormone deficiency resulting from a brain tumor. His parents are of average height. His predicted adult height without growth hormone (GH) treatment is approximately 160 cm (5 feet 3 inches). Billy is a short eleven-year-old boy with normal GH secretion according to current testing methods. However, his parents are extremely short, and he has a predicted adult height of 160 cm (5 feet 3 inches).[11]

Johnny's shortness is a function of disease and thus, on Daniels's account, deserves treatment. Billy, however, has a normal genotype, one that produces normal levels of GH. Thus Billy's shortness is not a function of disease, and on Daniels' account does not deserve treatment.

While Johnny and Billy are different with respect to GH secretion, they are similar in that both will suffer equally from being short in a culture that values tall stature. Thus one might ask, does the treatment/ enhancement distinction obscure our responsibility to respond to the suffering of both—regardless of the fact that one has a disease and one is healthy? Assuming for the purposes of argument that GH would be equally effective in both cases, would we make a mistake if we said that giving GH to Johnny would be a treatment, but giving it to Billy would be an enhancement?

While Daniels acknowledges that this is a hard case, he argues that his normal function model remains the best alternative for those trying to articulate a basic package of health care. In the end, he reminds us that his model assumes that different individuals have different capabilities and traits. The purpose of medicine is not to eliminate all differences. Rather, it is to restore people "to the range of capabilities they *could be expected to have had* without disease or disability" (p. 124), given their draw in the so-called natural lottery. Thus while Johnny and Billy are a hard case for those who in general are committed to responding to suffering, treating Johnny and Billy as the same would produce a still larger problem. Treating them the same would entail undermining our fundamental commitment to preserving differences, to promoting the health of populations made up of people whose normal function takes different shapes. If we abandoned Daniels's account of the proper purposes of health care, he argues that we would have to accept the still more problematic aspiration to level all differences to the extent that we can. At least for many who reject the aspiration to level such differences, Daniels's argument is persuasive.

There is another problem with the normal function version of the treatment/enhancement distinction, which Eric Juengst raises,[12] for which there may not be as clear a response as there was to Allen and Fost's. The normal function account runs into conceptual trouble when it is applied to "a limitlessly beneficial personal enhancement like moral sensitivity, intellectual acumen, or social grace." Juengst points out that on Daniels's own account, the notion of species-typical functioning is not merely a statistical notion, but implies a *theoretical* account of the design of the organism (that describes the "natural functional organization of a typical member of the species"). Juengst suggests that—*statistically*—it may be possible to draw out a spectrum of human psychosocial capacities, with an average middle term. *Theoretically,* however, it is very difficult to know what species-typical moral sensitivity, intellectual acumen, or social grace is. Thus, the species-typical functioning account doesn't provide definitive guidance in those cases where we are talking about the prospect of enhancing such capacities. And thus even if one accepts that the treatment/enhancement distinction is not arbitrary when it comes to some physiological functions like heart rate or growth hormone secretion rate, it is not easy to know how far the normal function model can get us with psychosocial functions like moral sensitivity or social grace.

There are not only problems with the intelligibility of the distinction itself. According to Anita Silvers, another problem with the distinction between treatment and enhancement is that it presupposes a notion of, and inadvertently valorizes, "the normal."[13] She suggests that the usual deployment of this distinction presupposes that to "promote equality of opportunity we must create a system *that restores inferior individuals to average competence.*" On her view, a commitment to equalizing opportunity through "normalizing the functionality of those who have disabilities" invites coercive and costly practices. One can read Norman Daniels's account of the importance of species-typical functioning upon which her argument depends differently from the way she does, and still accept the seriousness of the concern about the inadvertent valorization of "the normal." Indeed, in fairness to Daniels, it should be said that he is committed to trying to secure for individuals a range of opportunities, not to replicating specific forms of function—and not instead of securing better compensatory measures.

Nonetheless, it is important to grant the possibility that the treat-ment/enhancement distinction and the conception of normality upon which it depends could be used for coercive purposes. That conception of normality was in fact used, for example, when people who were post-polio were forced to use braces so that they could approximate "normal function"—rather than allowed to use (what in most cases would have been far more helpful) wheelchairs. But to grant this possibility suggests that we need to be on guard against this pernicious use of the distinction; it does not foreclose using it altogether.

There are at least two more important problems that will attend any attempt to employ the treatment/enhancement distinction to de-scribe the proper domain of medical practice and/or insurance reim-bursement. The first is that any individual's or any group of individuals' attempt to articulate a distinction like the treatment/enhancement one will, like all distinctions, take on a life of its own—regardless of the care with which someone like Daniels lays it out. Whereas Daniels employs the distinction with a view to providing people with what they need (a basic package of care), David Frankford's fundamental worry is that it will be used to keep people from getting what they need.

Frankford suggests that "students of public policy have long known that policy is rarely implemented as formulated."[14] The danger of a group such as ours making a policy statement about any version of the treatment/enhancement distinction is that, to begin with, "a statement that formulates a treatment/enhancement distinction potentially makes that distinction 'real.' " The problem with such a distinction becoming "real" is that it will mesh all too well with our current discourses about health policy, which "stress technical efficiency, and technical efficiency as a means to increase the size of the overall pie: the greatest goodies for the greatest number—utilitarianism (but nothing like sophisticated hybrid consequentialist models that attempt to account for distributive concerns)." That is, a version of the treatment/enhancement distinction like Daniels articulated in the hopes that it might do work in a sophisti-cated consequentialist scheme might in fact be appropriated by others and used for purposes very different from those intended by him. No matter how much we hope that we can specify our concerns about distributive justice, and no matter how much we specify our understand-ing of the tentative and problematic nature of the terms *treatment* and *enhancement*, they will be wrenched from the context in which we have articulated them.

In spite of his profound reservations about the uses to which the distinction will be put, Frankford acknowledges that it is already part of our "intersubjective use." This notion leads him to suggest that the way to minimize the potential for abuse is to try to limit our employment of the distinction to our conversations with medical professionals. Different from insurers, who on his view will surely tear the distinction from its "ethical moorings" and sweep it "into a sea of cost containment," he hopes that the distinction might be more thoughtfully used by medical professionals, who, as practitioners of "the art of the particular," attend to particularity and context. He concludes, "administration of a treatment/enhancement distinction in professional practice stands a much greater chance of being highly contextualized and incorporating all of cognitive, aesthetic, and ethical practical knowledge, than would administration of the distinction in the 'policy' world of contracts and health insurance."

Even if, in the age of managed care, one is skeptical about how clear the distinction is between insurers and medical professionals, Frankford's fundamental worry about the distinction being used to keep people from getting what they need will not go away. Whoever wants to wield the distinction needs to be committed to fighting the sorts of abuses he fears.

Last but not least, there is another practical difficulty with Daniels's view that the normal function version of the treatment/enhancement distinction can be used to help articulate a basic package of care. Assuming that one of the reasons we like the treatment/enhancement distinction is that it helps us to articulate such a package, it will be important to remember the following problem. The distinction does not square perfectly with current insurance practices that many of us take to be just nor will it square perfectly with what many of us would take to be a basic package of care. As Dan Brock points out, some *treatments* (for example, autologous bone marrow transplants for metastatic breast cancer) are not now covered by some insurance plans because they are deemed experimental and not cost effective.[15] Further, much insurance *does* cover some services that are *not* treatments, such as abortion. Finally, on Brock's account, some *enhancements are* covered by insurance because they prevent disease (for example, vaccination "enhances" normal immune system function). Parenthetically, as I mentioned above, it seems to me that it is not helpful to refer (as Brock does here) to vaccinations as enhancements; such interventions would fall directly into the *prevention* category if we could agree that we need a third category in addition to treatment and enhancement.

Regardless of where one comes out on the prevention question, it is clear that there is neither a perfect match between treatment and what insurance does or should pay for, nor between enhancement and what insurance does not and should not pay for. The absence of such a perfect match is a limitation for those who want to use the distinction as one part of their attempt to define a basic package of care.

In sum, like most distinctions, the treatment/enhancement distinction is fraught with problems. If, however, we recognize these problems, then we can use the distinction as one way *to begin* conversations about what doctors should and shouldn't do and what just systems of health care should and shouldn't reimburse. But as the foregoing discussion of the conceptual and practical problems suggests, it would be a mistake to think that it will be possible in some straightforward manner to read off the distinction itself what we should and shouldn't do. There is a big difference between hoping that a given distinction can begin conversation, and thinking it can end one.

In the current context, where there are financial incentives to provide fewer services, recognizing these problems should make us wary of decisions to refuse services based on the distinction. At the same time, critics of such cost savings should realize, as does Kathy Davis in her contribution to the collection,[16] that a nuanced conception of the distinction could in principle be used to help us begin to identify what we owe to each other. It could be one tool used to say what is and isn't included in a basic package of care.

### The Schmocter Problem

So far I have said how the treatment/enhancement distinction tends to be used by those who want to identify the proper goals of medicine— and ultimately the proper constituents of a basic package of health care. I have also identified several problems associated with that goals of medicine approach and the normal function model upon which it depends. But even if the normal function model and the treatment/ enhancement distinction were without limitations, even if we could clearly identify the important exceptions and caveats to the rule that medicine is only for the sake of treatment, we still would not yet have the theoretical resources we need to deal with concerns about what I have previously called the goals of society.

To appreciate this point, imagine for a moment a group of people who call themselves *schmocters,* a term coined by my friend and former colleague James Lindemann Nelson.[17] Schmocters don't claim to practice medicine. They widely advertise that they practice *schmedicine.* That is, they are expert in using new biotechnologies to enhance human capacities and traits, and they sell their expertise to willing, indeed, enthusiastic purchasers. Like some plastic surgeons today, these schmocters of the future don't rely on insurance reimbursement to make a living. More than enough people are eager to buy their services. Thus, even if talk about the "goals of medicine" could dissuade *doctors* from providing some services on the grounds that they are enhancements, and even if insurers refused to reimburse "enhancement" services, there is no good reason to think that *schmocters* would be dissuaded from providing those services. By definition, schmocters don't care about the goals of medicine, they care about the goals of schmedicine. The argument that appeals to the goals of medicine to shore up a prohibition of *doctors* pursuing enhancement would not suffice to prohibit *schmocters* from pursuing the same.

## Enhancement and the Goals of Society

Thus while the treatment/enhancement distinction makes sense in the context of the goals of medicine conversation, it does not make sense in another sort of conversation. And that is the sort of conversation that we will increasingly have to have: one about what we might call the goals of society. In this sort of conversation, one can't argue against a particular intervention on the grounds that it is not a treatment or not consistent with reasonable insurance practice. The problem is harder. In this sort of conversation, if one wants to claim that a given "improvement" will in some contexts be problematic, then one will have to argue that it is inconsistent with or undermines some important social value or goal. And that is a difficult sort of argument to wage.

It is important to notice just how disinclined many of us are to take such an argument seriously. Such disinclination is often articulated in variations on what I will here call the arguments from precedent. The conclusion of those arguments is that wariness about the prospect of aiming new technologies at enhancement is a familiar but unfortunate form of anxiety that does not deserve to be taken seriously. I will try to show that one of the problems with those arguments is that they do not appreciate the moral difference that new biotechnological means can make.

### Means Matter Morally

To begin with, means make an obvious moral difference when a given socially valued activity is predicated upon their use. As Dan Brock puts it in his contribution to the project, "In many valued human activities, the means of acquiring the capacities required for the activity are a part of the very definition of the activity, and transforming them transforms, and can devalue, the activity itself." Even when two different means are "in themselves" morally unproblematic, one means might not be a part of the definition of the activity, and thus using it would undermine the activity. For example, using a memory-enhancing drug might be morally unproblematic as a means to increase one's capacity to memorize poetry; but using the same means to gain an advantage in a chess match would be problematic insofar as the institution of chess does not allow for such means in its self-definition.[18]

But means can also make a moral difference in less obvious ways. As I have already noted, there is something indeed odd in worrying about aiming technologies at the "enhancement of human capacities." What after all is worrisome about improving a human capacity? Because enhancing human capacities is taken to be a fairly self-evident good, worries about it are often dismissed as being a function of unnecessary anxiety or fear about the new.[19] The arguments used to dismiss such anxiety are variations on what I have called *arguments from precedent*.[20]

While the argument is never put in such explicit form, its implicit structure is something like this: We've always used means A to achieve end A; means B also aims to achieve end A; therefore means B is morally unproblematic. For example, we've always increased the teacher/child ratio and reduced class room size (means A) to enhance student performance (end A); Ritalin (means B) also aims to achieve enhanced student performance (end A); therefore using Ritalin is morally unproblematic.

There are at least two sets of problems with this tendency of thought or form of argument. The first has to do with treating different *means* as morally the same; the second has to do with treating different *ends* as morally the same.

The first problem with treating different means as morally the same is that doing so can entail ignoring the important fact that different means sometimes work on what might be called different "objects." To use the previous example, whereas means A (increasing the teacher/

student ratio and reducing class size) changes the child's environment to enhance student performance, means B (Ritalin) changes the child's *biology*. While doing the former is not self-evidently any more morally unproblematic than the latter is problematic, different means obviously will produce different sorts of experience for the child; at a minimum, one experience entails taking medication and the other entails learning with fewer classmates; one experience entails reduced "noise" in the child's brain, the other reduced noise in her classroom.

Indeed, some new means that work on our bodies instead of our environments may incline us to ignore the complex social roots of the suffering of individuals. And the easier it is to change our bodies to relieve our suffering, the less inclined we may be to try to change the complex social conditions that produce that suffering. As new biotechnological means enable us to respond to suffering that results when some humans are subjected by others to hostile and unfair conditions (such as overcrowded classrooms and overheated markets), we must be careful to attend to the difference that means can make.

Another problem with this version of the argument from precedent, intimately related to the first, is that it ignores the fact that different means can embody and/or express different values. For example, in her essay, "Aspirin for the Mind? Some Ethical Worries about Psychopharmacology," Carol Freedman compares Prozac and talk therapy as different means aimed at relieving psychical pain.[21] According to Freedman, whereas the psychopharmacological means are embedded in a mechanistic conception of the self, talking therapy is embedded in a much different and richer conception. As she puts it, what is at stake in how we treat psychical pain "is a conception of ourselves as responsible agents, not machines." On this view, if we think that emotional problems are rooted in our interpretations of our experience, then, as animals capable of insight,

> we should have a basic commitment to addressing those problems with insight and understanding. Otherwise, we are not respecting what it is to be a self. For central to maintaining the idea of a self is the commitment to regard some of our actions and attitudes as justified by our reasons, not explained in mechanistic terms.

To give up the idea that sometimes we act based on our reasons and interpretations would be to give up the idea that we are responsible for what we do. Opting only for the pharmacological, mechanistic response lends itself to our thinking of ourselves more and more in mechanistic terms—and less and less in terms of being responsible agents. Thus the argument from precedent can sometimes obscure the difference that a given means makes for how we think about and value ourselves.

Arguments from precedent can also obscure the fact that different means can produce *ends* that appear to be the same, but in fact are the same with respect to only one measure. As Ron Cole-Turner points out, while prayer and Prozac may both increase serotonin levels, the end-states achieved by those different means are only the same with respect to that one measure.[22] We are mistaken to assume that the ends at which the means aim are equivalent in all morally significant ways.

Intimately related to that problem is another. Arguments from precedent can also mistakenly assume that the ends are relevantly similar when in fact the magnitude of the change effected by the two means is radically different. That is, these arguments can ignore the moral difference that the magnitude of the change achieved by the new means can make. It is true, for example, that humans have for a long time tried to shape their progeny. Enhancement germ-line engineering is "just like" matchmaking in that the end of both "procedures" is to influence the shape of offspring. But to say that the procedures are morally the same requires ignoring that they achieve results with vastly different degrees of precision. The degrees of precision are so different that they are arguably different in kind. Again, while this difference does not say that the more precise procedure is morally problematic,[23] it does suggest that we should attend to the difference that magnitude can make—as well as attend to the respects in which ends that appear to be "the same" are not.

In sum, we must be wary of arguments that too quickly assume or assert that the means—or ends—are "just the same" as the older and accepted ones. To say that the "new" means or ends may be different in ways that matter morally does not require us to defend the view that the new means or ends are unique. Just as there are probably no uniquely new social and ethical problems, there are probably no uniquely new means or ends. The issue for us is to try to get better at discerning how "new" means or ends exacerbate "old" social and ethical problems.

Three primary areas of social and ethical concern were identified in the course of our project: unfairness in the distribution of resources; complicity with suspect norms; and inauthenticity and threats to self-understanding.

## Concerns about Unfairness

In a recent editorial in *Science*, "Science in the 21st Century," President Clinton identified "four guideposts" that our country needs to remember if we are going to put new scientific knowledge to good rather than evil purposes.[24] The very first guidepost is the following.

> [S]cience and its benefits must be directed toward making life better for all Americans—never just a privileged few. Its opportunities and benefits should be available to all. Science must not create a new line of separation between the haves and the have-nots . . . (p. 1951).

President Clinton's words suggest the obvious but profound problem raised by aiming new biotechnologies at the enhancement of human capacities. Those who already have economic resources will readily gain access to new technologies, and those new technologies will make them stronger competitors for more resources. Imagine a new drug or genetic technology that enabled us to sleep less and thus be more productive. Presumably, those who had access to the technology would, as a result of their newfound productivity, win more resources. Those without the resources to purchase the new technology would be that much farther behind.

Parenthetically, we should note that it is logically possible that all members of our society might gain access to the same technology, thereby providing no competitive or positional advantage to anyone. Given the current situation in the United States, however, where there is not even universal access to treatment, the chances of universal access to enhancements (with significant financial costs) seem rather dim. But if there were universal access to enhancement, then we would be faced with what Dan Brock calls "self-defeating enhancements." If everyone achieved the same relative advantage with a given enhancement, then ultimately no one's position would change; the "enhancement" would have failed if its purpose was to increase competitive advantage.

Back in the "real world" of U.S. public policy, some will surely ask, Why shouldn't new science and technology make life better "for only a privileged few"? Isn't that what new science and technology have always done? This form of the argument from precedent is as regularly invoked as it is corrupt. There are many things that we've always done that we think we ought not to do either now or in the future. Exploiting and oppressing others are two.

Moreover, as suggested above, it is naïve to believe that all new biotechnologies are just more of the same. To make that point, perhaps it is useful to make a crude distinction between purchasing new tools and purchasing new capacities. In the past the rich have had access to new technological tools that enabled them to increase their productivity and thus their resources. Access to the tool that is the printing press, for example, no doubt conferred a competitive advantage on those who could afford access to it and its products. But how much one could benefit from those new tools and products was to some extent limited by one's draw in the genetic lottery. (It goes without saying that how much one could benefit was also limited by other things, like one's upbringing.) If one got a "good genetic draw" and was good at using printed materials, then presumably one would prosper better than somebody else with the same genetic draw but without access to those products. One of the new things about the new biotechnologies is that one's draw in the genetic lottery does not pose the same sort of limitation. Now, in addition to buying access to the new technologies (like print), we have the prospect of people purchasing, as it were, a better genetic draw. Thus having resources makes one a doubly strong competitor for new resources. Again, the distinction between purchasing new tools and purchasing new capacities is crude and definitely *not* an argument for never letting individuals purchase new capacities. But bearing the distinction in mind may help us resist those arguments from precedent that are waged to dismiss concerns of the sort articulated by President Clinton.

From a public policy point of view, it is unfortunate that even if we were all persuaded that some enhancement technologies ought not to be for sale on the grounds that they would confer an unfair competitive or positional advantage, a significant problem would remain. As Dan Brock has pointed out, in many real cases "enhancements will in part confer competitive or positional advantages on those who obtain them, *but in part also constitute intrinsic goods that confer noncompetitive benefits.*"[25] Brock gives the example of a drug that improves concentration. Presumably, such a drug could confer both a competitive benefit (one would be better able to concentrate and thus better able to perform on everything from taking tests to betting on the market) and also confer a noncompetitive benefit (one would be better able to concentrate and thus enjoy Shakespeare or Schubert). As Brock puts it, "The complexity for public policy would be that concerns about fairness . . . would support some limits on the use of this enhancement, but these limits would at the same time be criticized as denying individuals the possibility of gaining significant, intrinsic benefits."

To a reluctant consequentialist like myself, the notion of "*intrinsic benefits*" is not transparent. Even though I am somewhat skeptical about the suggestion that some people will purchase biotechnological enhancements because they want the "intrinsic benefit" of reading Shakespeare (as opposed to the extrinsic benefit of reading Shakespeare faster so that they can perform better on tests and thus ultimately in the market), I take Brock's point. The argument will be made that these technologies are desired not only because they provide a competitive advantage, but because they are good in themselves. How to adjudicate such questions will be one of the harder problems for policymakers in this arena.

While concerns about distributive justice are profoundly important, our project spent relatively little time on them. Those who want to think more about distributive justice and unfairness would do well to start with Maxwell Mehlman and Jeffrey Botkin's *Access to the Genome: The Challenge to Equality* (Georgetown University Press, 1997).

## Concerns about Complicity

A considerable amount of our group's energy was spent thinking about the problem of what Maggie Little called "complicity with harmful conceptions of normality" (where by "normality" she refers not to any putatively value-free biological notion but rather to an altogether value-laden cultural notion).[26] It was during our exploration of cosmetic surgery that we got the clearest idea about how certain enhancements might exacerbate the problem of complicity with such conceptions. That exploration entailed attempts to understand the extent to which we are free to avail ourselves of biotechnologies that relieve our individual suffering; the extent to which our choices to use those technologies are constrained by social forces; and the extent to which we are responsible to criticize and resist using those technologies that relieve the suffering of individuals (on the grounds that they reinforce or are complicit with the social forces that create that suffering).

One of Kathy Davis's great contributions was to show the respects in which women's choices to undergo cosmetic surgery are free and that such surgery is often undertaken to relieve real suffering. Though her focus is indeed on women's agency, she never forgets the extent to which women are constrained in their decisions to change the shape of their bodies. She observes,

> Women's relation to their appearance is constrained by cultural definitions of feminine beauty. Cosmetic surgery can only be a viable option in a context where medical technology makes the surgical alteration of the body both a readily available and a socially acceptable solution to women's problems with their appearance. Women's willingness to calculate the risks of surgery against its benefits can only make sense in a context where a person is able to view her body as a commodity, as a possible object for intervention—a business venture of sorts.[27]

But rather than emphasize the need to remove or transform those constraints, Davis explores how, within those constraints, "cosmetic surgery enable[s] women to become embodied subjects rather than objectified bodies" (p.161). That is, Davis stresses the extent to which, with a view to relieving their own suffering, women freely choose to reshape their bodies. "For a woman whose suffering has gone beyond a certain point, cosmetic surgery can become a matter of justice—the only fair thing to do" (p. 163).

One of Susan Bordo's crucial contributions to our project was to show and emphasize the extent to which women's choices to avail themselves of "enhancements" are constrained.[28] Bordo spends as much time and energy attending to the social forces exerted on women as Davis spends on their decisionmaking processes. In particular, Bordo focuses on the forces exerted by the images that the movie and advertising industries create to sell their products. Alluding to the movie *Braveheart* and the shoe company Nike, Bordo nicely sums up her critique:

> The worst thing, in the *Braveheart*/Nike universe of values, is to be bossed around, told what to do. This creates a dilemma for advertisers, who somehow must convince hundreds of thousands of people to purchase the same product while assuring them that they are bold and innovative individualists in doing so. The dilemma is further compounded by the fact that many of these products perform what Foucault and feminist theorists have called "normalization." That is, they function to homogenize our diversity and perpetuate social norms, often connected to race and gender. This happens not necessarily because advertisers are consciously trying to promote racism or sexism, but because in order to sell products they have to either exploit or create a perception of personal *lack* in the consumer. . . . An effective way to make the consumer feel inadequate is to take advantage of values that are already in place in the culture. For

example, in a society where there is a dominant (and racialized) preference for blue-eyed blondes, there is a ready market for blue contact lenses and blonde hair-coloring. The catch is that ad campaigns which promote such products also re-glamorize the beauty ideals themselves. Thus they perpetuate racialized norms.

Bordo shows the extent to which advertisers teach us what our conceptions of ourselves and our life projects ought to be. She thinks that Davis is mistaken about the extent to which we are free to choose what to do with our bodies. "There is a consumer system operating here, which depends upon our perceiving ourselves as defective, and which will continually find new ways to do this. That system—and others which are connected to it, generating new technologies and areas of expertise organized around the diagnosis and correction of 'defect'— is masked by the rhetoric of personal empowerment."

Again, whereas Davis attends to cosmetic surgery as a means with which women can relieve their own suffering, Bordo attends to it primarily as a source of suffering. "Cosmetic surgery is more than an individual choice; it is a burgeoning industry and an increasingly normative cultural practice. As such, it is a significant contributory *cause* of women's suffering, by continually upping the ante on what counts as an acceptable face and body."

If we are going to take seriously the respects in which our actions are and are not free, the extent to which our life projects are and are not our own, and the extent to which we must hold ourselves and each other responsible for the values propagated by our uses of new biotechnologies aimed at "enhancement," then it would help to begin thinking more in terms of what Maggie Little calls an *ethics of complicity*. While Little's discussion grows out of reflections on enhancement and the *doctor-patient* relationship, it can also help us think about the *schmocter-consumer* relationship. That is, even if we had no worries about how a given enhancement might undermine or violate the goals of medicine, we would still be concerned that it would promote complicity with harmful societal conceptions of normality. Whether doctors or schmocters are the providers, what is crucial is the relationship of the "providers" and "consumers" to the system of norms that the enhancement aims to fit.

But let us begin where Little does, with a description of the "suspect system" of norms and practices with which both physicians and patients can be complicit. To help characterize that system, Little provides examples that help to distinguish among "levels" of suspect norms.

For her first example, she imagines a society in which people with voluptuous chins are the dream Saturday night date. According to Little's analysis, the suffering that goes with not having such a chin is due to attitudes that are unfortunate but not unfair. She suggests that, "while we may pity [the distress of the person with the paltry chin] and empathize with his misfortune, we should not regard it as a pain that implicates society."[29]

Her next two examples, however, do implicate society. The first involves a boy who is not just not asked out on dates, but is ostracized because his ears stick straight out. "Here the costs imposed for such deviation [from society's norms]—the teasing, the ostracism—are grossly out of proportion to society's own reflective valuation of the norm. They are punitive, intolerant, in a word, cruel." Different from the first case, at work here is not a preference, but a prejudice.

The third example involves a black person who requests to become more white and a woman who requests to make her body's shape more like Barbie's. Little argues that while the cruelty associated with such norms is part of what is immoral about the third case, that is not all. The further source of "social culpability" is that the very norms of appearance at issue are "morally suspect." She writes, "We feel a special heightened moral unease about these cases . . . because the norms of appearance at issue are grounded in or get life from a broader system of attitudes and actions that are in fact *unjust*." For African-Americans to want to become more white is not "some aesthetic whimsical prefer- ence." It is a function of an ugly history in which being black is devalued and being white valorized. Similarly, changing the shape of women's bodies is situated in a particular and hurtful history. Again, we are talking about sufferings that are due, not to some departure from species-typical functioning, but rather to "some attitude or practice of society that is morally troubling." We are talking about sufferings due to norms whose content "is steeped in injustice."

Little asks one of our group's fundamental and vexing questions: When is it acceptable to accommodate these pressures? It's very nice for academics to observe that an individual's suffering has complex social and historical roots, but what difference should that make to a suffering individual—or to a surgeon—who has at hand means to relieve that suffering? What should an individual do—or what should a surgeon do—who doesn't have the time to wait for those complex social and historical roots of the suffering to whither?

In the end, Little's answer is that, to the extent that one's actions do (or can reasonably be seen to) endorse or promote norms that undergird a system of unjust practices and attitudes, one is obliged elsewhere to fight that same system. Little suggests that both the patient who avails herself of the technology and the physician who supplies it take on the responsibility. One might understand a reluctant act of complicity to be the best alternative response to a given form of suffering. But then one should be all the more energized to fight that same system in other contexts and at other times. While Little's response may not be tidy, it has the virtue of attending both to the fact that sacrificing individuals on the altar of social change can be unjust—and to the fact that the one who makes such accommodations has the responsibility to find other opportunities to fight the social system that produces that suffering.

There is of course a respect in which Little's analysis does not apply to *schmocters*. It might not make sense to require *schmocters* to help their clients to decide whether they are culpable in their choice to get, say, cosmetic surgery. As Dan Brock has quipped, asking *schmocters* to engage in the sort of self-exploration Little recommends might be a bit like asking car salesmen to explore with customers the virtues of mass transit. But even if one cannot hope that *schmocters* will help promote education of the sort that Little's analysis calls for, one can hope that policymakers at other levels will consider how to promote such education. Just as potential patients and physicians need to consider the extent to which their actions are complicit with such hurtful conceptions of normality, so must policymakers and consumers more generally.

## Concerns about Inauthenticity

One of our project's primary case studies was what Peter Kramer has called "cosmetic psychopharmacology"—that is, psychopharmacology used not to treat disease, but to shape personality in "attractive" ways.[30] Prozac was one of the key examples of cosmetic psychopharmacology, and the one to which Carl Elliott's work was devoted.[31] Elliott wondered whether some "improvements" of the sort described by Kramer might ultimately undermine one fundamentally valuable sort of life project. Elliott asked Kierkegaard's famous question, the one so many of Walker Percy's novels explore: "Suppose we could relieve all of us of our sense of spiritual emptiness or alienation, of our feeling of being disoriented and lost in the world. Would that be a good thing? Or is it sometimes better to feel bad than to feel good?" He elaborates:

> Suppose you are a psychiatrist and you have a patient [whose alienation is caused by his recognition that all of his beliefs and practices are up for

grabs]; say, an accountant living in Downers Grove, Illinois, who comes to himself one day and says, Jesus Christ, is this it? A Snapper lawn mower and a house in the suburbs? Should you, his psychiatrist, try to rid him of his alienation by prescribing Prozac? Or do you secretly think that maybe, as bad off as he is, he is better off than his neighbors? Because even though he's in a predicament, at least he's aware of it, which is a lot better than being in a predicament and thinking you're not.

Why might anyone object to relieving real suffering if the means are at hand? Elliott suggests that if you want to answer that question you need to grasp two features of what he, following Lionel Trilling and Charles Taylor, calls an *ethics of authenticity*. First, you need to notice that many of us think of our lives as a project. The notion of life as a project depends upon the idea that "the sense or significance of our lives depends on how we live them." And that idea in turn depends upon the idea that to some extent our lives "are planned undertakings which, to a large extent, we control and for which we are responsible."[32] The second feature of the ethics of authenticity that we need to grasp is that to answer the question, How should I live? one has to look inward. "You have to be true to yourself."

But with the aspiration to authenticity comes the possibility of inauthenticity, the possibility of not leading one's own life. On Elliott's account, the fear of such inauthenticity motivates much of the concern about drugs like Prozac. Prozac may relieve my unhappiness, but it is *my* unhappiness. It is the unhappiness into which I have grown, and it is the unhappiness with which I want to make my peace. "It would be worrying if Prozac altered my personality, even if it gave me a better personality, simply because it isn't *my* personality."[33]

Whereas many Americans are committed to the idea of *authenticity*, it may be that many more of us are committed to the related but distinct idea of *self-fulfillment*. As Weber argued in *The Protestant Ethic and the Spirit of Capitalism,* for those who live in Luther's wake, work takes on a moral character. It becomes a calling. Not being devoted to it is a moral failing. And as Elliott observes, this idea gets played out in interesting ways in America. "What Luther referred to as a calling [to God] survives nowadays . . . as a calling from within: the idea of discovering yourself, of finding your own particular place in the world. A meaningful life . . . is something that you discover and create on your own, *especially through the life of work and the life of family and household*" (emphasis added).

While Elliott entirely appreciates the virtues of this worldview, he observes that for many of us it comes to mean that if we are not aggressively pursuing prosperity and happiness with the fervor urged by our founding fathers, then we are letting ourselves down and squandering our time on earth. Given that many of us Americans feel it is our duty to pursue self-fulfillment and happiness on the Weberian model, it would not be surprising if many of us came to feel it our duty to use any means possible to fulfill it—including taking drugs like Prozac. (Note that we're *not* talking here about using drugs like Prozac to treat clinical illness.)

For those committed to the idea of *authenticity*, using drugs to pursue the idea of *self-fulfillment* is disturbing. That of course is not the ground for an outright prohibition of the use of such drugs for such purposes. But appreciating that drugs like Prozac are good at promoting self-fulfillment as opposed to authenticity is useful if one wants to remember that such drugs are not "all purpose means." These drugs are not good for simply any life project. They are good for a particular sort of life project.

To Peter Kramer's credit, he is acutely aware of, and writes about, the extent to which Prozac might be seen to promote the "virile values" of a capitalist society. Yet in the end Kramer stands by his claim that Prozac is a "feminist drug," which, when prescribed by a wise doctor and in conjunction with talk therapy, can be used by women (and men) to promote whatever life projects they see as fit. To make vivid what he has in mind when he speaks of the wise doctor who can help his patients pursue whatever life project they want, he invokes the image of Dr. Yang in Woody Allen's movie *Alice*. In invoking Dr. Yang and Alice, Kramer seems to forget what life project Alice decides to pursue after she is aided by the wise doctor and his drugs. Different from nearly all of Kramer's patients, who become better at pursuing the sort of life projects currently valorized by our culture, Alice rejects those projects and that culture. With Mother Teresa as her model, Alice gives up her life of unfettered consumption, and commits herself to a life of poverty and charity.

We are so deeply embedded in our own way of life that many of us find it impossible to imagine that it is a very particular kind of life. If we value critiques of and departures from those conceptions of the "normal life project," then we are going to have to get much better at noticing when a drug is promoted as being good for any life project, but is in fact good for only one (albeit widely acclaimed) sort. Inauthenticity is not a new problem, created by technologies aimed at the enhancement of human capacities. But with the power of these new pharmaceuticals comes the potential to exacerbate that old problem.

Whereas Elliott was concerned that certain "enhancements" might promote a turning away from a form of anxiety or feeling bad that is constitutive of a life lived courageously and authentically, project participants like Gerald McKenny and Mary Winkler were concerned that some "enhancements" might promote a turning away from the vulnerability, imperfection, and finitude that is constitutive of life altogether. As Gerald McKenny puts it, "To the extent that enhancements overcome, or lead us to deny, the vulnerability of the body, they also foreclose the kinds of self-formation that our awareness of vulnerability makes possible."[34] Along similar lines, Mary Winkler argues that our advertising practices reveal the depth of our desire to gain control over what, ultimately, is beyond our control: the fact of our own finitude.[35] That is, our desire for control and stability put us at risk for missing what Winkler calls our "full humanity." We risk forgetting that we are ultimately and essentially vulnerable creatures.

While McKenny and Winkler both worry that "enhancement technologies" may promote our tendency to forget or ignore what sort of creature we really are, neither of them thinks that such a worry should preclude our taking seriously the desire for "enhancements." As Winkler generously puts it, when talking somewhat skeptically about some cosmetic surgeries, "I would not ignore the desires of any—they are all human desires."

Surely the sorts of turning away from fundamental life experiences worried about by Elliott, McKenny, Winkler, and others, are not new. Inauthenticity is not a new problem, created by aiming biotechnologies at the enhancement of human capacities. Though inauthenticity may not be a new problem, it is one that new "enhancements" have the potential to exacerbate.

## Considerations for Public Policy

If the deliberations of the project working group did not lead to specific policy recommendations, they did make clear the considerations that are essential for thoughtful policymaking with regard to the use of new technologies to "enhance" human capacities and traits.

*It would be a mistake to think that the treatment / enhancement distinction will ever provide good, transparent moral guidance* about the particular decisions faced by individuals such as doctors or institutions such as managed care companies. The distinction should not be looked to for transparent guidance about whether a doctor should use a given means to relieve a given individual's suffering—or about whether a managed care company should provide such means. Like many distinctions, the treatment/enhancement distinction is permeable, unstable, and can be used for pernicious purposes. If used carefully, however, it can be one tool to start important conversations about the sorts of health care services that a just system of health care should provide.

*It would be a mistake to think that the new biotechnologies are just more of the same.* We should give up the arguments that take the form, "we've always done it." It is true that we have always sought enhancement. But arguments from precedent glibly excuse us from thinking about how new means to achieve old ends make a moral difference. Worrying about technologies aimed at the enhancement of human capacities and traits is not the same as worrying about apple pie.

*The term* enhancement *can alert us to and start conversations about the potential for exacerbating long-standing problems* such as unfairness, complicity, and inauthenticity.

- We must all become cognizant of the fact that "enhancements" have the potential to widen the gap between the haves and have nots. Making policy in light of that concern will always be made difficult by the fact that some of the new biotechnologies will offer both a competitive advantage and a noncompetitive (or "intrinsic") advantage. A drug that could truly enhance memory is an example of such a biotechnology. In spite of that difficulty, it will be extremely important for policymakers to become increasingly aware that these new biotechnologies have the potential to widen the gap to an unprecedented extent. Further research is needed to come up with strategies to avoid putting new biotechnologies to purposes that will widen the already huge gap between the haves and have nots.
- We must all become vigilant about knowing when new "enhancements" are complicit with harmful conceptions of normality. The enormous problem here is that it requires understanding our motivations as consumer-citizens. When are we availing ourselves of a biotechnology because we have been duped by a dominant norm, and when are we availing ourselves of it because we're trying to play with the system or enter that system to change it? Research is needed to create educational strategies that would enable individuals to engage in the sort of self-exploration that could help them reach decisions about "enhancements" in a more truly informed way.

While some forms of enhancement in some contexts may obviously be problematic, many more will not be. As long as we are committed to relieving suffering, and such technologies are a means to do that, we will always have good reason to employ them. The great challenge is to find ways to relieve such suffering that do not perpetuate harmful conceptions of normality. The challenge is to learn simultaneously to attend to the suffering of individuals and to criticize and resist the systems that produce that suffering.

• We must all become vigilant about noticing that whereas many new biotechnologies will be marketed as "all purpose means," they may not be. Many will be good only for one currently valorized but narrow sort of life project. Even if there were nothing wrong with the dominant conceptions of a good life that reign in our culture today, there would be something wrong with pretending that those are the only worthy conceptions—or that the means which advertisers want to sell us are "good in themselves." Further research is needed to develop strategies to provide individuals with opportunities to recognize the difference between means that are truly "all purpose" and ones that are just advertised that way.

Finally, I would advise that those who follow our project into the enhancement fields take on smaller and more manageable parcels of it. Our colleagues at Case Western Reserve University's Bioethics Center, for example, are limiting their study to genetic enhancement. We here at The Hastings Center would like to study the even narrower question concerning the "enhancement" uses to which the new "antidepressants" are being put. Not only should smaller cases be taken on, but smaller policy questions need to be tackled in greater depth. We hope that our project has done some of the conceptual ground clearing that will make it easier for others to toil in these fields.

### Acknowledgments

This essay was written with generous support from the National Endowment for the Humanities (RH-21271-95). It was first published as a special supplement to volume 28, no. 1 (1998) of the *Hastings Center Report*. I gratefully thank the following people for reading and commenting on earlier versions of this essay: Erika Blacksher, Dan Brock, Carl Elliott, David Frankford, Eric Juengst, Margaret Olivia Little, Carol Tauer, and Robert Wachbroit. Needless to say, the remaining mistakes and infelicities are mine alone.

## NOTES

**1.** In a thought experiment, LeRoy Walters and Julie Gage Palmer ask this question. See *The Ethics of Human Gene Therapy* (New York: Oxford University Press, 1997), pp. 126–27.

**2.** NEH Grant number RH-21271-95.

**3.** James E. Sabin and Norman Daniels, "Determining 'Medical Necessity' in Mental Health Practice," *Hastings Center Report* 24, no. 6 (1994): 5–13, at 5.

**4.** Norman Daniels, "The Genome Project, Individual Differences, and Just Health Care," in *Justice and the Human Genome Project*, ed. Timothy F. Murphy and Marc A. Lappe (Berkeley: University of California Press, 1994), pp. 110–32, at 122.

**5.** Sabin and Daniels, "Determining 'Medical Necessity,' " p. 10.

**6.** Daniels, "The Genome Project, Individual Differences, and Just Health Care," p. 122.

**7.** Sabin and Daniels, "Determining 'Medical Necessity.' "

**8.** For alternative versions of the distinction, see Eric Juengst, "What Does *Enhancement* Mean?" this volume.

**9.** Walters and Palmer, *Ethics of Human Gene Therapy*, pp. 110–11.

**10.** See Eric Juengst, "Can Enhancement Be Distinguished from Prevention in Genetic Medicine?" *The Journal of Medicine and Philosophy* 22, no. 2 (1997): 125–42; Juan Manuel Torres "On the Limits of Enhancement in Human Gene Transfer: Drawing the Line," *The Journal of Medicine and Philosophy* 22, no. 1 (1997): 43–53.

**11.** Cited in Daniels, "The Genome Project," p. 123.

**12.** Juengst, "What Does *Enhancement* Mean?"

**13.** Anita Silvers, "A Fatal Attraction to Normalizing: Treating Disabilities as Deviations from 'Species-Typical' Functioning," this volume.

**14.** David Frankford, "The Treatment/Enhancement Distinction as an Armament in the Policy Wars," this volume.

**15.** Dan Brock, "Enhancements of Human Function: Some Distinctions for Policymakers," this volume.

**16.** Kathy Davis, "The Rhetoric of Cosmetic Surgery: Luxury or Welfare?" this volume.

**17.** Nelson credits Saul Kripke's discussion of identity (and "shmidentity").

**18.** See Thomas H. Murray, "Drugs, Sports, and Ethics," in *Feeling Good and Doing Better: Ethics and Nontherapeutic Drug Use*, ed. Thomas H. Murray, Willard Gaylin, and Ruth Macklin (Clifton, New Jersey: Humana Press, 1984); Peter J. Whitehouse et al., "Enhancing Cognition in the Intellectually Intact: Possibilities and Pitfalls," *Hastings Center Report* 27, no. 3 (1997): 14–22.

**19.** John Harris, *Wonderwoman and Superman: The Ethics of Human Biotechnology* (New York: Oxford University Press, 1992); Henry I. Miller, "Gene Therapy for Enhancement," *The Lancet* 344 (1994): 316–17; Dorothy C. Wertz, "Society and the Not-So-New Genetics: What Are We Afraid Of?" *Journal of Contemporary Health Law and Policy* 13 (1997): 299–346.

**20.** Erik Parens, "Should We Hold the (Germ) Line?" *Journal of Law, Medicine & Ethics* 23, no. 2 (1995): 173–76.

**21.** Carol Freedman, "Aspirin for the Mind? Some Ethical Worries about Psychopharmacology," this volume.

**22.** Ronald Cole-Turner, "Do Means Matter," this volume.

**23.** Indeed, one might well argue that reaching an acceptable aim with greater precision is, all other things being equal, better.

**24.** Bill Clinton, "Science in the 21st Century," *Science* 276 (1997): 1951.

**25.** Brock, "Enhancements of Human Function."

**26.** Margaret Olivia Little, "Cosmetic Surgery, Suspect Norms, and the Ethics of Complicity," this volume.

**27.** Kathy Davis, *Reshapng the Female Body: The Dilemna of Cosmetic Surgery* (New York: Routledge, 1995), p. 157.

**28.** Susan Bordo, "*Braveheart, Babe,* and the Contemporary Body," this volume.

**29.** Little, "Cosmetic Surgery, Suspect Norms, and the Ethics of Complicity."

**30.** Peter D. Kramer, *Listening to Prozac* (New York: Viking, 1993).

**31.** Carl Elliott, "The Tyranny of Happiness: Ethics and Cosmetic Psychopharmacology," this volume.

**32.** See also, Carol Freedman, "Aspirin for the Mind?"

**33.** This issue is complex. Dan Brock asks: If features of my personality with genetic causes are mine, why aren't features caused by Prozac—if it is I who took the drug with the intention of producing those features?

**34.** Gerald McKenny, "Enhancements and the Ethical Significance of Vulnerability," this volume.

**35.** Mary Winkler, "Devices and Desires of Our Own Hearts," this volume.

ERIC T. JUENGST

# *What Does* Enhancement *Mean?*

The term *enhancement* is usually used in bioethics to characterize interventions designed to improve human form or functioning beyond what is necessary to sustain or restore good health. Understood in this way, enhancement functions as an important concept in two different moral conversations: the discussion of the proper limits of biomedicine, and the discussion of the ethics of self-improvement.[1] These two conversations are overlapping, but the enhancement concept plays quite different roles in each. Furthermore, there are a number of different interpretations of the enhancement concept alive in the literature, which vary in their ability to play these different roles. For policymakers faced with the prospect of using enhancement as a regulatory concept, it will be important to have a clear map of these uses and interpretations, and that is what this essay attempts to provide.

## *Two Uses of* Enhancement

In discussions of biomedicine's domain, enhancement usually functions as a moral boundary concept. Just as the concept of futile treatment is used to indicate the limits of medicine's obligations to perform interventions with diminishing power to achieve any medical goals, "enhancement" is typically used to mark the limits of professional obligations to pursue biomedical interventions that can achieve goals beyond medicine's. Like futile treatments, enhancement interventions fall outside of medicine's proper domain of practice: patients have no role-related right to demand them of the profession, and physicians who do provide them bear a burden of justification for doing so that does not apply to medically necessary interventions. By extension, the enhancement boundary concept can be called upon to help define the social role of the medical profession, demarcate the proper sphere of biomedical research, and help set limits on health care payment plans. *Enhancement* helps us frame the proper domain for biomedicine in these contexts

*Thrus. May 10th 3:50 #13*

by providing a conceptual cap for the enterprise in an era when its technological capacities seem to have fewer and fewer upper limits.

When it is used as a boundary concept, enhancement, like futility, plays both descriptive and normative roles. We need to be able to identify the boundary when we encounter it—to be able to identify our efforts as either futile or enhancing—and we need to know what the boundary implies for our professional obligations to continue. For futile interventions, these two roles are nicely congruent: interventions are futile when they no longer work, and when they no longer work they are no longer required. For enhancement interventions, however, the descriptive and normative implications of calling them "enhancements" seem to be at cross purposes. While futile treatments literally do no good, enhancements are by definition and description improvements: changes for the good. Yet, normatively, the function of calling them "enhancements" is to place them beyond the pale of proper medicine. For a profession dedicated to pursing the improvement of its patients, the fact that enhancements act, descriptively, just like all the other improvements the profession strives to achieve makes it difficult to discern when an intervention transgresses the normative boundary that the concept purports to mark. Thus, while all useless interventions count as "futile," it becomes necessary to specify what kinds of improvements count as "enhancements" in order to apply the concept. This need has provoked a number of different interpretations of the enhancement concept, tailored to different biomedical boundary-drawing problems.

In discussions of people's personal decisions to improve themselves or their children, enhancement plays a different role. Here, the concept functions normatively like the concept of paternalism. It does not mark a clear moral watershed, since we can think of many examples in which the behavior it refers to is morally justified and even obligatory. But the concept does indicate the questions that one should ask of situations to which it applies. Thus, while to identify paternalism in a situation does not settle the matter morally, it does suggest that we should be careful to ask questions about coercion, decision-making capacity, and levels of benefit.[2] Identifying enhancement in a case of personal decision-making functions similarly to indicate the range of relevant moral questions to pose against the circumstances at hand. In these discussions, enhancement is less a boundary marker than a signpost, allowing travelers to orient themselves within the several moral boundaries relevant to their location. This orientation makes it possible to judge the ethics of personal and parental practices, and, by extension, to develop public policies regulating enhancement that are independent of the rules that regulate biomedicine.

As different line-drawing problems in medicine have generated different substantive interpretations of the enhancement boundary concept, so different moral concerns about personal improvement have provoked different accounts of the background issues to which the enhancement signpost should point us. Here again the use of the concept is shaped by the fact that, in most circumstances, the personal improvement of ourselves and our children is morally laudable. The reasons why a particular improvement will count as a morally suspicious enhancement will always depend upon the goals and values of the human activity that provides the scale against which the improvement is measured, rather than on some intrinsic feature of the intervention itself. Different spheres of activity will produce different accounts of what an ethically problematic improvement looks like and the background questions it raises.

It is confusing enough that the concept of enhancement means different things to different moral wanderers, relieving physicians of the need to go further and reminding parents of the dangers that lie ahead. But the different accounts of the marker itself—the interpretations of what counts as an "enhancement," how we know one when we see one, and what specific moral hazards it signifies—create another layer of complexity. Like all locals, the bioethicists who inhabit this murky country are happy to provide directions to travelers, and usually do so in terms of their own local landmarks—the interpretations of "enhancement" that are most suited to the specific issues they address— regardless of whether these interpretations will help the travelers get to their specific destinations. The next two sections attempt to catalog these local versions of the enhancement concept, and to suggest the implications of each as either a boundary concept for medicine or a signpost for the rest of us.

## Enhancement as Opposed to Treatment

One common way of describing enhancement is by exclusion: enhancement interventions are any interventions designed to produce improvements in human form or function that do not respond to legitimate medical needs. This approach interprets enhancement as one side of a distinction, and seeks to use an independent account of its opposite—"treatment"—to explain how enhancement interventions differ from the forms of human improvement we do accept as medically necessary.

However, making the distinction between treatment and enhancement is not without complexities. The distinction is explicated in three distinctly different ways, which have different merits as either boundary markers or moral signposts. There are accounts that turn on the concept of disease, accounts that use medicine's professional goals, and accounts that rely on theoretical measures of "species-typical functioning" that go well beyond medicine.

## Disease-based Accounts

Probably the most common way to explain the distinction between treatment interventions and enhancement interventions is to distinguish the problems to which they respond. Treatments are interventions that address the health problems created by diseases and disabilities— "maladies" in the helpful language of Clouser, Culver, and Gert.[3] Enhancements, on the other hand, are interventions aimed at healthy systems and normal traits. Thus, prescribing biosynthetic growth hormone to rectify a diagnosable growth hormone deficiency is legitimate treatment, while prescribing it for patients with normal growth hormone levels would be an attempt at "positive gene therapy" or enhancement.[4] On this account, to justify an intervention as appropriate medicine means to be able to identify a pathological problem in the patient; if no medically recognizable malady can be diagnosed, the intervention cannot be "medically necessary," and is thus suspect as an enhancement.[5]

This interpretation has the advantages of being simple, intuitively appealing, and consistent with a good bit of biomedical behavior. Maladies are objectively observable phenomena and the traditional target of medical intervention. We can know maladies through diagnosis, and we can tell that we've gone beyond medicine when no pathology can be identified. Thus, the pediatric endocrinologists discourage the enhancement uses of biosynthetic growth hormone by citing the old adage "If it ain't broke, don't fix it."[6] This interpretation is also the one at work in the efforts of professionals working at the boundary, like cosmetic surgeons, to justify their services in terms of relieving "diagnosable" psychological suffering rather than satisfying the aesthetic tastes of their clients, and in our insurance companies' insistence on being provided with that diagnosis before providing coverage for such surgeries.

But this interpretation also faces at least two major difficulties. The first problem is the problem of prevention. While efforts at generic "health promotion" straddle the border of biomedicine, efforts to prevent the manifestation of specific maladies in individuals are always accepted as legitimate parts of biomedicine and are automatically located on the "treatment" side of the enhancement boundary. On the other hand, one of the ways one can prevent a disease is to strengthen the body's ability to resist it long before any diagnosable problem appears. These forms of prevention all attempt to "fix" bodily functions that aren't "broken," and thereby seem to slide into enhancement. Consider the case that LeRoy Walters and Julie Palmer make for including some genetic enhancements within the domain of legitimate medical needs. They start with the paradigm of a nongenetic preventive intervention— immunization against infectious disease—and then drive their genetic truck through the border-crossing it creates:

> In current medical practice, the best example of a widely-accepted health-related physical enhancement is immunization against infectious disease. With immunizations against diseases like polio or hepatitis B, what we are saying is in effect, "The immune system that we inherited from our parents may not be adequate to ward off certain viruses if we are exposed to them." Therefore, we will enhance the capabilities of our immune system by priming it to fight against these viruses.
>
> From the current practice of immunizations against particular diseases, it would seem to be only a small step to try to enhance the general function of the immune system by genetic means. . . . In our view, the genetic enhancement of immune system function would be morally justifiable if this kind of enhancement assisted in preventing disease and did not cause offsetting harms to the people treated by the technique.[7]

One gene therapy protocol already under way "treats" people with an inherited high risk of heart disease by increasing the number of low density lipoprotein receptors their blood cells carry, enhancing their ability to clear high levels of cholesterol from their blood before it causes heart disease.[8] If it works to reduce their risk of heart disease, why not use it prophylacticly to reduce my more modest risk? But if protocols like these are acceptable as forms of preventive medicine, how can we claim that we should be "drawing the line" at enhancement?[9]

One response to the problem of altering healthy traits to help prevent disease is to point out that the intervention is performed, like treatment, with the intent to control objective disease and that intent is proved by the fact that we deem such interventions failures if their target malady occurs, regardless of what other improvements they might provide.[10] This response, of course, only can reassure us about the use of those interventions that fail. It means giving, for example, a cognitive enhancement intervention that claims to prevent Alzheimer's disease (while making you smarter) the advantage of the man who claimed his dance was keeping dragons out of Central Park: until a dragon lands it is hard to argue that he's not providing a preventive service.

The second problem that any disease-based interpretation of the enhancement boundary faces is, of course, biomedicine's infamous noso-logical elasticity. It is not that hard to coin new maladies for the purposes of justifying the use of enhancement interventions.[11] By interpreting the boundary of medicine in terms of maladies, this approach puts the power for drawing that boundary squarely in the profession's hands, with the corresponding potential for abuse.

### Ideological Accounts

A second approach to interpreting the enhancement/treatment distinction begins by taking the last point to heart and extrapolating from it. If there is no objective way to identify and describe medical maladies and distinguish them from psychosocial problems (like racial stigmatization or aesthetic discrimination), then perhaps the enhancement/treatment distinction itself is best understood as a social construction reflecting the medical profession's current values and willingness to perform interventions across different cases.[12] Under this view, medicine really has no proper boundaries, and practitioners and their patients should be free to decide together what problems to count as "diseases" and what interventions to count as "treatments."

This view resonates well with a number of contemporary social scientific critiques of biomedicine.[13] It also provides a simple normative lesson for professionals concerned about their obligations in specific cases: One takes one's cues from the patient's value system, and negotiates toward interventions that can help achieve the patient's vision of human flourishing. However, it does fail to satisfy in one important respect: it makes the enhancement concept and the enhancement/treatment distinction useless in trying to articulate the limits of medicine and "medical necessity" for policy purposes. To the extent that useful "upper-boundary" concepts are required at the policy level—for societies making health care resource allocation decisions outside the market system, for example—this impotence is an important weakness.

### Normalcy Accounts

The last major approach to interpreting the treatment/enhancement distinction is often framed explicitly in terms of the need for a policy tool that can separate legitimate health care needs from luxury services. One of the most developed expositions of this third view is Sabin and Daniels's endorsement of what they call the "normal function" standard for determining the limits of "medically necessary" (and therefore socially underwritten) mental health services.[14]

Sabin and Daniels agree with the skeptics that it is not necessary, and probably fruitless, to try to draw a conceptual line between legitimate treatment and nonmedical enhancements by trying to distinguish their objects as disease entities or degrees of positive health. Instead, they argue that an appropriate line can be drawn simply by thinking about how to provide medical services fairly within a population. Following Daniels's earlier work, they construe health care as one of society's means for preserving equality of opportunity for its citizens, and define health care needs as those services that allow individuals to enjoy the portion of the society's "normal opportunity range" to which their full array of skills and talents would give them access, by restoring or improving their abilities to the range of functional capacities typical for members of their reference class (e.g., age and gender) within the human species. Daniels has specified this definition of health care needs further by saying that the notion of "species-typical functioning" it relies upon is not "merely a statistical notion," but implies "a theoretical account of the design of the organism," that describes the "natural functional organization of a typical member of the species."[15] Any interventions that would expand an individual's range of functional capacities beyond the range typical for his or her reference class would count as an (medically unnecessary) enhancement. Thus, Sabin and Daniels write:

> Treating illness and enhancing human capabilities may both be desirable social goals, but they should not be confused with one another. The normal function model holds that health care insurance coverage should be restricted to disadvantages caused by disease and disability unless society explicitly decides to use it to mitigate other forms of disadvantage as well.[16]

The "normal function" approach is a sophisticated attempt to define the limits of social obligations to provide health services for policy purposes, and comes close to accurately reconstructing the rationale behind many actual "line drawing" judgments by health care coverage plans and professional societies. Unfortunately, this approach is also semipermeable in an important way for our purposes.

The normal function interpretation runs into trouble when applied to the problem of a limitlessly beneficial personal enhancement like moral sensitivity, intellectual acumen, or social grace. Two of Sabin and Daniels's weakest assumptions betray it: that we have a "theoretical account of the design of the organism" robust enough to specify "species-typical function" in these areas, and that an individual's "skills and talents" are fixed as a base-line constraint on the available opportunity range by the "natural lottery" of human genetics.

On the first score, what do our theoretical accounts of human personal traits suggest about their "species-typical" functioning? Statistically, of course, it is possible to draw out a spectrum of human psychosocial capacities, with an average middle range: a "norm" in the empirical sense that Daniels rejects as inadequate for his purposes. But "theoretically"? Contemporary human biology, set as it is within the context of modern biology generally, admits of very few open-ended functional goals in our organismic design beyond reproductive fitness. But in fact, we humans often allow the spread of our "memes" to take precedence over the spread of our genes. Just as some plants can never live too long, and some animals can never have too many offspring, humans can never seem to have too much intellectual, moral, or spiritual experience. Or at least if there is an optimum level of experience in those spheres, biological theory is not the place to turn to in seeking to define it.

The second problem of the "opportunity range" account in trying to deal with personal enhancements is a problem of fairness that flows directly from our inability to discern the "optimum" level for improvements in these traits.

Sabin and Daniels assume that people's "talents and skills" (read: psychosocial capacities) are inborn, largely immutable, and most often unequal. Since they are (correctly) committed to the idea that "the general principle of fair equality of opportunity does [should] not imply leveling individual differences,"[17] their vision of fair access to health care would yield a system in which every individual could have the services needed to realize his or her "full array" of personal talents and skills, regardless of the resulting disparities.

But if everyone's talents and skills can themselves be improved, it becomes difficult to resist an "equalizing" policy that would discriminate against the naturally fortunate. If a statistical norm is used as a goal for services, then all those born above the norm will be denied access. If the ceiling was set at the level of the species' psychosocial champion, the less fortunate would have a disproportionate claim on enhancement resources. To those, like Daniels, who value the ability of each individual, including the champions, to realize the "full array" of opportunities he or she can reasonably achieve, such a claim to extra enhancement resources by the unfortunate would also be an unfair claim, and thus a bad way to define the limits of acceptable enhancement practices.

Finally, it should be apparent that, in any of its forms, attempting to define enhancements by contrasting them with legitimate medical treatment can only be of limited value to individuals and parents concerned about the ethics of personal improvement. To know that a particular improvement is not medically indicated, or a job for doctors, or even biologically normalizing does raise some base-line ethical questions for individuals and parents: Are there health risks involved? Can I trust the "schmoctors" who do provide the service?[18] Do I hold beliefs that prohibit me from ever aspiring to be better than average? Since most applaud human efforts to surpass some species-typical norms, and are happy to work with professionals outside of medicine to achieve that end, and are even willing to accept some level of health risks for themselves and their children in the process, this kind of signpost, if it is the only one used by policymakers, is not likely to provide much guidance to the perplexed. The answers to questions at this level, which are usually already stipulated or assumed in our conversations about the ethics of personal improvement, pale in comparison to some set of real issues, which this approach to enhancement cannot raise. If policymakers seek an account of enhancement that can serve as both boundary maker and moral signpost, they will need to look further.

## Enhancement as Opposed to Achievement

Indeed, our conversations about the ethics of self-improvement do tend to be dominated by a second major approach to interpreting enhancement. Here, the defining feature of a morally suspicious enhancement intervention is interpreted to be the nature of the means used to achieve a given improvement, rather than whether or not the intervention is deemed "medically necessary." There are several ways in which this concern for means is explicated. Among those interested in the ethics of self-improvement, many argue that, quite apart from any health risks, some means of personal self-improvement—exercise, education, prayer—are "natural" to their goals while "artificial" approaches—drugs, surgeries, implants—are simply not. Personal improvements should be earned by discipline and effort, the argument goes, and to acquire them through biomedical interventions is to cheapen their value and cheat the social practices in which they play a role. At the extreme, acquiring improvements through genetic enhancement interventions may reflect hubris on our part; an attempt to "play God" in a blasphemous way. Those involved in discussions of performance-enhancing drug use in sports have called this view "pharmaceutical Calvinism"[19] to highlight its emphasis on a work ethic, but suitably broadened (as "biomedical Calvinism"?), it also serves nicely to capture these critics' concerns about interfering in God's genetic plan for the world.

### Enhancements as Artificial

There are several threads in this argument that should be untangled. One sometimes sees in this view a form of naturalism: that the pharmaceutical shortcut to happiness is wrong because it is "artificial," while traditional means of improvement like exercise, prayer, and education are acceptable because "natural." For theological writers, the distinction is often grounded in (or refuted by) views of the proper relation of humans and God: to use biomedical means to improve ourselves is to "play God" in a dangerously overreaching way. It risks hubris in a way that humbly accepting the limits of natural achievement does not.[20] For the psychologically minded, the "natural" means to improvement are sometimes interpreted as more "authentic" means, and therefore preferable to artificial interventions that would mask or devalue the true nature or identity of the person improved.[21] For those within religious traditions that draw clear lines between the proper domains of human and divine action, or for those with a clear commitment to a particular form of personal authenticity, these naturalistic interpretations of the distinction may serve as useful moral signposts. But outside those private spheres, it is hard to operationalize this naturalism for public policy purposes. What should the state make of this claim in which educational regimens, religious rituals and the conventions of sports are playing the role of the "natural," while empirical observations, biological materials and organic chemicals are labeled as "artificial"?

### Enhancements as Corrosive Shortcuts

Fortunately, the other threads in the argument over whether means matter in understanding enhancement are stronger. The first focuses on the idea that biomedical enhancements, unlike achievements, are a form of cheating. This view assumes that taking the biomedical shortcut somehow cheats or undercuts the specific social practices that would make the analagous human achievement valuable in the first place. Thus, some argue that it defeats the purpose of the contest for the marathon runner to gain endurance chemically rather than through training, and it misses the point of meditation to gain Nirvana through psychosurgery. In both cases, the value of the improvements lie in the achievements they reward as well as the benefits they bring. The achievement—successful training or disciplined meditation—add value to the improvements because they are understood to be admirable social practices in themselves. Wherever a corporeal intervention is used to bypass an admirable social practice, then the improvement's social value—the value of a runner's physical endurance or a mystic's visions—is weakened accordingly. If we are to preserve the value of the social practices we count as "enhancing," it may be in society's interest to impose a means-based limit on biomedical enhancement efforts.[22]

Interpreting enhancement interventions as those which short-circuit admirable human practices in an effort to obtain some personal goal has special utility at two levels of ethical analysis. First, for individuals, it highlights the challenge that enhancement poses to their moral integrity: to what extent can they take credit for their accomplishments if they do not achieve them through the socially valued practices that have traditionally produced them? This question is not one about either causation or responsibility: clearly, they are still the authors of their accomplishments. It would be a mistake for the student whose Ritalin-induced concentration yields a high exam grade from one night's cramming to think that it was literally the Ritalin that took the test and made the grade. The question is whether the student earned the grade; that is, whether the grade is serving its usual function of signaling the disciplined study and active learning that the practice of being a student is supposed to involve. If the grade is not serving that function then, for that student, it is a hollow accomplishment, without the intrinsic value it would otherwise have.

Moreover, this interpretation of enhancement also has implications for the policies of the social institutions that maintain the practices we value. To the extent that biomedical shortcuts increasingly allow specific accomplishments, like test-taking, to be divorced from the admirable practices they were designed to signal, the social value of those accomplishments will be undermined. Not only will the intrinsic value be diminished for everyone that takes the shortcut, but the resulting disparity between the enhanced and unenhanced will call the fairness of the whole game (be it educational, recreational, or professional) into question. If the extrinsic value of being causally responsible for certain accomplishments is high enough (like professional sports salaries), the intrinsic value of the admirable practices that a particular institution was designed to foster may even start to be called into question. For institutions interested in continuing to foster the social values for which they have traditionally been the guardians, this argument has two alternative policy implications. Either the institutions must redesign the game (e.g. education or sports) to find new ways to evaluate excellence that are not affected by available enhancements, or they must prohibit the use of the enhancing shortcuts. Which route an institution should take depends on the possibility and practicality of taking either, because ethically they are equivalent.

As useful as this means-oriented interpretation of enhancement is at pointing out potential moral dangers to individuals, parents, and institutions, it has a limited value in helping physicians define the bounds of legitimate medicine. Concerns over the authenticity of their patients' achievements or the corruption of social practices might deter some physicians from prescribing performance-enhancing drugs, but only as a matter of personal, not professional conscience. Like parents trying to use the treatment/enhancement distinction as a guide, the enhancement/achievement distinction only serves to mark the most basic considerations for physicians contemplating simple physical enhancements: does this intervention cheat some practice in any way that has already been explicitly forbidden by society (i.e., is it legal?). There is one way in which this understanding of the enhancement problem can provide a boundary marker for medicine, however, and that is by asking whether a given intervention actually short-circuits or undermines the physician's own sphere of practice: namely, his or her commitment to the welfare of the patient.

It is in the form of the latter question that this understanding of the enhancement problem is most often invoked in the biomedical literature, because this question does provide one way to tell when one has hit a medical boundary. Bodily improvements are all self-limited by the basic design requirements of the human body. For any particular bodily part or process, "improvement" will pass through an optimal point of peak benefit, after which its further pursuit would be increasingly detrimental to the body as a whole. Thus, the cholesterol-dredging efficiency of blood cells can be improved by increasing their LDL receptors, but after a point that would in turn produce a deficit of cholesterol harmful to the nervous system. This optimizing quality makes it significantly easier to tell when one has gone too far with an intervention, and suggests comfortably familiar normative lines to draw: when an intervention no longer optimally benefits the body by biomedical criteria, it should be forgone and refused.

### Enhancement as a Perversion of Medicine

Unfortunately, some of the social games we can play (and cheat in) do not turn on participants' achievements at all, but on traits over which individuals have little control, like stature, shape, and skin color. The social games of stigmatization, discrimination, and exclusion use these traits in the same manner that other practices use achievements: as intrinsically valuable keys to extrinsic goods. Now it is becoming increasingly possible to seek biomedical help in changing these traits in order to short-circuit these games as well.[23] Here, the biomedical interventions involved, like skin lighteners or stature increasers, are "enhancements" because they serve to improve the recipient's social standing, but only by perpetuating the social bias under which they originally labored. Any normal medical tool that cured one patient by making other patients' problems worse would be considered medically perverse, and in this case the perversion is compounded by the fact that the problem in question is social, not somatic. When *enhancement* is understood in this way, it warns of still another set of moral concerns.

On this interpretation, what makes the provision of human growth hormone to a short child a morally suspicious enhancement is not the absence of a diagnosable disease or the dictates of medical policy or the "species atypical" hormone level that would result: rather it is the intent to improve the child's social status by changing the child rather than by changing her social environment. This interpretation of the enhancement concept carries heavy prescriptive messages for both professional practice and personal conduct. Enhancement interventions are almost always wrongheaded under this account, because the source of the social status they seek to improve is, by definition, the social group and not the individual. Attempting to improve that status in the individual without regard for its social nature amounts to a moral mistake akin to "blaming the victim": it misattributes causality, is ultimately futile, and can have harmful consequences. This interpretation of enhancement seems to be at work when people argue that it inappropriately "medicalizes" a social problem to use Ritalin to induce cooperative behavior in the classroom or that breast augmentation surgery only exacerbates society's sexist vision of beauty.[24] In each case, the critics dispute the assumption that the human need in question is one that is created by, and quenchable through, our bodies, and assert that both its source and solution really lie in quite a different sphere of human experience.[25]

This interpretation of the enhancement concept is useful to those interested in the ethics of personal improvement because it warns of a number of moral pitfalls beyond the base-line considerations that the enhancement/treatment distinction provides. Attempting to improve social status by changing the individual risks being self-defeating (by exacerbating the individual's sense of inadequacy by inflating expectations), futile (if the individual's comparative gains are neutralized by the enhancement's availability to the whole social group), unfair (if the whole group does not have access to the enhancement), or complicitous with unjust social prejudices (by forcing people into a range of variation dictated by biases that favor one group over others). For those faced with decisions about whether to use performance-enhancing drugs in sports or to insert the "leadership gene" into their embryos, this way of understanding enhancement is much more illuminating than attempts to distinguishing it from medical treatment.

For policymakers interested in using enhancement as a regulatory concept, on the other hand, this interpretation of the enhancement concept does have one drawback. Under this interpretation, enhancement interventions are biomedical interventions which (mistakenly) attempt to improve a patient's social characteristics. More often than not, however, such interventions will be understood by those who accept them as "treatments" for legitimate medical problems: for example, the psychological distress of being socially unsuccessful. This move opens the door for the significant cross-talk that one finds, for example, in the literature on the ethics of cosmetic surgery, between those critics who apply the enhancement concept to point out the moral dangers of self-improvement, and those advocates who sidestep the warning by using the enhancement/treatment distinction to argue that no enhancement is involved in their practice. In these situations, it may make better sense to forgo the enhancement concept altogether, and use another broader concept, like "medicalization," to refer to the mistake of applying the medical model to the wrong problems.

The medicalization of social problems, as opposed to merely assisting patients to cheat in specific social achievements, also has significant implications for the boundaries of medicine. While stature or speed can at least be measured by medicine, there is a large class of traits— loyalty and competitiveness, leadership and stewardship, aggression and altruism, for example—that cannot even be perceived without a larger frame of reference. These latter are all traits that characterize our interactions with and evaluation by other people: the machinery of social flourishing. In fact, they are traits that are impossible to identify or evaluate without reference to the social context of the individuals who display them: the solitary shipwreck survivor does not display them. Thus, the improvement of these traits has traditionally been the domain of our social engineers: teachers, ministers, coaches, and counselors, supported by policymakers charged with creating environments in which such traits can be cultivated. When attempts are made to shift the improvement of these traits into the domain of the doctor, by working directly on the substrates for social capacities that our bodies provide, medicine runs up against a basic epistemic boundary. It is not clear how one would identify any optimum or even maximum conditions for social traits through medical means alone.[26] For example, what dosage of human growth hormone will insure optimum social advantage? This question suggests a test for one kind of enhancement boundary: if criteria drawn from other spheres of experience seem like better measures of improvement than medical measures, then the intervention in question should probably count as an *enhancement* that goes beyond medicine's domain of expertise. Because of its own epistemic limits, the argument goes, biomedicine should restrict its ambitions to the sphere of bodily dynamics, which it knows something about, and leave the sphere of social dynamics in the hands of the other human values specialists: parents, educators, preachers, counselors, accountants, and coaches.[27]

## Conclusion

Clearly, all of the ways of understanding "enhancement" as a moral concept that I've reviewed have limitations. However, all these interpretations do seem to be alive and well and mixed together in the literature on the topic. That may be part of the reason why the normative implications of transgressing the "enhancement" boundary have never been entirely clear. For example, while the futility debate asks whether medically futile interventions are ever professionally permissible, the ethical questions of the enhancement debate range much more widely: Enhancement interventions are not "medically necessary," but we seem unsure whether such interventions should be considered "contraindicated" as professional practices, or whether they are ethically neutral options "electable" by patients, or whether they can ever be prescribed, even if safe and efficacious, as a valid health service. Before we can decide, we need to know which version of "enhancement" we are using in any given policy discussion.

As I have shown, it is not possible to cleanly assign the different interpretations of *enhancement* to different spheres of ethical analysis. But some rough correlations might be made. Thus, the interpretation of "enhancement" in terms of the enhancement/treatment distinction seems most useful where it is the limit of medicine's expertise that is at issue. Whether medicine's boundary is defined in terms of concepts of disease, or in sociological terms as the scope of medical practice, or in terms of some theory of the human norm, this interpretation at least provides tools to draw that boundary. Moreover, all other considerations being equal, the line that it draws is the boundary of medical obligation, not the boundary of medical tolerance. Using this tool, enhancement interventions like cosmetic surgery can still be permissible to perform as physicians, but also permissible to deny. This interpretation has important implications for social policymaking about health care coverage to the extent that society relies on medicine's sense of the medically necessary to define the limits of its obligations to underwrite care. Again, all other considerations being equal, this interpretation of the concept suggests that few enhancement interventions should be actively prohibited by society or forgone by individuals, even when they are not underwritten as part of health care, since there is nothing intrinsically wrong with seeking self-improvements beyond good health.

By contrast, the interpretations of enhancement that focus on the misuse of biomedical tools in efforts at self-improvement seem the most relevant to issues in the personal, rather than professional, ethics of enhancement. Concerns about the authenticity of particular accomplishments are moral challenges to the individual, but find little purchase in the professional ethics of biomedicine, with its focus on the physical safety and efficacy of its tools. The primary policy implications of this interpretation are for the social institutions charged with fostering particular admirable practices: enhancement interventions that offer biomedical shortcuts to achievement force reassessments within those institutions of the values they stand for and the practices they have designed to foster them.

Finally, at the other end of the spectrum, enhancement interventions that seem to commit the moral mistake of trying to address social problems through the bodies of the potentially oppressed do seem to mark a stronger set of moral boundaries for all concerned. For biomedicine, this concept marks an epistemic limit beyond which medical approaches to problem-solving are not only unnecessary but conceptually wrongheaded. For individuals, parents, and society, these kinds of enhancement interventions risk either back-firing by exacerbating the social problems they are intended to address, or being futile if they merely result in a shift of the normal range for a given social trait. Where the medicalization account of enhancements fits a given intervention, there does seem to be more justification for stronger warnings, protections, or prohibitions across the board, whether the intervention falls within medicine's boundaries or not.

## Acknowledgment

This paper has been made possible by grants from the National Endowment for the Humanities to The Hastings Center (RH-21271-95), and from the National Institute for Human Genome Research to Case Western Reserve University (R01-HG01446), and by the able assistance of two research assistants: Erica Wagner, and JaeHak Son.

## NOTES

**1.** I am grateful to Erik Parens for this idea regarding two different conversations, which he contributed to one of our many talks about these matters. He is not responsible, however, for the baroque superstructure which I have built upon it. Just cite it as "Erick's Enhancement Distinction" and we'll both be happy.

**2.** James Childress, *Who Should Decide: Paternalism in Health Care* (New York: Oxford University Press, 1982).

**3.** K. Danner Clouser, Charles Culver, and Bernard Gert, "Malady: A New Treatment of Disease," *Hastings Center Report* 11 (1981): 29–37.

4. Edward Berger and Bernard Gert, "Genetic disorders and the ethical status of germ-line gene therapy," *Journal of Medicine and Philosophy* 16 (1991): 667–85.

5. Norman Daniels, "Growth hormone therapy for short stature: can we support the treatment/enhancement distinction?" *Growth, Genetics and Hormones*, Suppl. 1, 8 (1992): 46–48.

6. Ad Hoc Committee on Growth Hormone Usage. "Growth hormone in the treatment of children for short stature," *Pediatrics* 72 (1984): 891–94.

7. Leroy Walters and Judy Palmer, *Ethical Issues in Human Gene Therapy* (New York: Oxford University Press) (forthcoming) chapter four, mss. pp. 13–14.

8. James Wilson et al., "Ex Vivo gene therapy for familial hypercholesterolemia," *Human Gene Therapy* vol. 3, no. 2 (1992): pp. 179–222.

9. W. French Anderson, "Human Gene Therapy: Why draw a line?" *Journal of Medicine and Philosophy*, 14 (1989): 681–93; Eric T. Juengst, "Can Enhancement be Distinquished from Prevention in Genetic Medicine?" *Journal of Medicine and Philosophy* 22 (1997): 125–44.

10. Eric T. Juengst, "Can Enhancement?" pp. 125–42.

11. Kathy Davis begins her book with the report of hearing a cosmetic surgeon justify a nose bob on a teenage Moroccan girl living in Holland as treatment for her "inferiority complex based on racial characteristics." Kathy Davis, *Reshaping the Female Body: The Dilemma of Cosmetic Surgery* (New York: Routledge, 1995), p. 2.

12. H. Tristram Engelhardt, "Persons and Humans: Re-fashioning Ourselves in a Better Image and Likeness," *Zygon* 19 (1984): 281–95. H. T. Engelhardt, "Human nature technologically revisited," *Social Philosophy and Policy* 8 (1990): 180–91.

13. J. Byron, *Good, Medicine, Rationality and Experience: An Anthropological Perspective* (New York: Cambridge University Press, 1994).

14. James Sabin and Norman Daniels, "Determining 'Medical Necessity' in Mental Health Practice," *Hastings Center Report* 24 (1994): 5–13.

15. Norman Daniels, *Just Health Care* (New York: Cambridge University Press, 1986).

16. Sabin and Daniels, "Determining Medical Necessity."

17. Daniels, *Just Health Care*, p. 33.

18. Erik Parens, "Is Better Always Good? The Enhancement Project," this volume.

19. Gerald L. Klerman, "Psychotropic Hedonism vs. Pharmacological Calvinism," *Hastings Center Report* 2, no. 4 (1972): 1–3.

20. Ted Peters, "'Playing God' and Germline Intervention," *Journal of Medicine and Philosophy* 20 (1995): 365–86.

21. See Jaquelyn Slomka, "Playing with Propranolol," *Hastings Center Report* 22, no. 4 (1992): 13–17.

**22.** Thomas Murray, "Drugs, Sports and Ethics," *Feeling Good and Doing Better: Ethics and Nontherapeutic Drug Use*, ed. T. Murray, W. Gaylin, R. Macklin (Clifton, N.J.: Humana Press, 1984): p. 107–29.

**23.** Erik Parens, "The Goodness of Fragility: On the Prospect of Genetic Technologies Aimed at the Enhancement of Human Capabilities," *Kennedy Institute of Ethics Journal* 5 (1995): 141–53.

**24.** Kathryn Morgan, "Women and the Knife: Cosmetic Surgery and the Colonization of Women's Bodies," *Hypatia* 6 (Fall 1991): 25–53.

**25.** Glenn McGee, *The Perfect Baby: A Pragmatic Approach to Genetics* (New York: Rowan and Littlefield, 1997).

**26.** W. French Anderson, "Human Gene Therapy: Why Draw a Line?" *Journal of Medicine and Philosophy* 14 (1989): 681–89.

**27.** Hans Jonas, "Biological Engineering—A Preview," *Philosophical Essays from Ancient Creed to Technological Man*, (Englewood Cliffs, N.J.: Prentice Hall, 1974), p. 140–41.

DAN W. BROCK

# Enhancements of Human Function: Some Distinctions for Policymakers

Human beings have always sought means of enhancing human capacities, and we now appear on the verge of greatly expanded abilities to do so. The Hastings Center project on technologies aimed at the enhancement of human capacities originally aimed to develop policy guidelines for such enhancements, and more specifically to elucidate the various factors that are relevant for determining appropriate policy responses for different enhancement technologies. The project focused on three case studies—cosmetic surgery, psychopharmacological engineering, and genetic engineering—but I shall not restrict my discussion to them because only by looking at a wide array of enhancements will we understand their full ethical and public policy complexities. One might hope that a relatively simple classification of enhancement technologies might be possible for the purposes of developing public policy guidelines for them. The main argument of this paper, however, is that no such simple classification or guidelines are possible because of several kinds of complexities which I will briefly explore, or at least illustrate, here.

First, there are too many different kinds of enhancements, which extend substantially beyond the three paradigm cases mentioned above; for example, many common activities of parents or social institutions are designed to enhance the capacities of individual humans, although we may not think of them as technologies, such as music lessons or sports camps for children. Second, too many different policy responses are possible to different enhancement technologies; for example, beyond simply prohibiting or permitting are a variety of ways of more or less strongly discouraging or encouraging the development and use of such technologies. Third, there are simply far too many morally important features of enhancement technologies, as well as moral considerations and arguments that bear on the appropriate policy responses to them.

The overall upshot of these complexities is that it is unrealistic to expect to develop any simple classification of different enhancement technologies, or guidelines for the development of appropriate public policy for them. My aim in this paper will be to try to bring out some of this complexity in the hope of making our thinking about public policy for human enhancement technologies more consistent, nuanced, and systematic. At this relatively early stage in thinking about public policy for new technologies like psychopharmocology and genetic engineering, the greatest danger may be to attempt to respond too quickly, unsystematically, and in ad hoc ways to different technologies as they gain public attention and concern, and thereby to miss some of the important considerations that make these policy issues so complex.

## *Moral Categories of Enhancements*

Before turning to the complexities of different kinds of enhancement technologies and policy responses to them, it is worth noting that within ethics itself, there are different moral categories into which different enhancement technologies can be placed. Use of some enhancements is widely believed to be morally required for the benefit of the individuals whose capacities are enhanced. Vaccines that are used to enhance individuals' responses to specific health threats, and which are typically required for children before they enter school are one example. Another example of a morally required enhancement activity, if not technology, is education itself; parents are legally required to send their children to school, or to develop alternative plans for their education at home, at least until the children reach age 16. This action is believed to be morally required in order to give children, and the adults they will become, the minimum skills necessary for a reasonable array of opportunities in life.

Use of another large category of enhancements is generally considered to be morally permissible, that is, neither morally required nor morally prohibited. Examples include parents providing music lessons for their children and individuals having cosmetic surgery; in both cases, most people believe that it should be up to the individual parents, or to the individuals considering cosmetic surgery, to decide whether to employ these enhancements.

Another moral category of enhancements includes those generally considered morally prohibited. Some people believe this category includes only enhancements used by one party for another party, while others believe that it also includes enhancements used by an individual for him or herself. For example, some people support prohibiting any use of enhancement technologies with a sufficiently poor risk/benefit ratio; other enhancements used by parents for their children should be morally prohibited if they come at the cost of violating the child's right to an open future, a case to which I shall return later.

The moral categories into which different enhancements can be placed are, of course, more complex than this simple three-part classification; for example, what may be most important about some enhancements is their relationship to the development of specific moral virtues, such as compassion or benevolence, or their impact on important social values such as community.

## Different Kinds of Policy Responses
## to Enhancement Technologies

Just as there are a variety of moral categories that can be applied to different enhancement technologies, there is also a broad range of possible public policy responses to various enhancement technologies. In illustrating some of these different responses, I shall assume that it is the state, that is, the government in some form and at some level, that is setting policy. However, public policy is not made only by direct state action. At least quasi-public policy is also made by a variety of nongovernmental institutions. For example, a variety of professional bodies in medicine have substantial influence over medical practice through promulgation of a variety of regulations and guidelines. To the extent that government permits, authorizes, or even enforces these regulations, they constitute at least de facto public policy, even if the government does not itself promulgate the regulations and guidelines. But even if we focus only on direct governmental action, there is a wide range of policy responses that represent sometimes subtly different attitudes, evaluations, and regulations of different enhancement technologies.

There is a continuum of positive and negative governmental responses to different enhancement technologies. At the mid-point of this continuum is complete neutrality—a "hands off" policy in which government takes no action that significantly affects the development or use of the technology. The continuum extends in both positive and negative directions from this mid-point, and I will first explore the positive end. Government can encourage the use of enhancement technologies in a variety of ways without directly supporting them or requiring their use; for example, government can support or carry out educational programs to encourage parents to get their children vaccinated to enhance the capacity of their children's immune systems to ward off disease. These attempts at persuasion leave others free to accept or reject the intended influence of the persuasive programs. Government can provide additional support for enhancement technologies like vaccines by providing financial incentives or support for the development of such vaccines, for example, through research support from the National Institutes of Health. Incentives can also be provided to individuals to make use of these enhancement technologies once they are developed, such as subsidies to parents of the costs of vaccinating their children.

Moving from persuasive to coercive interventions, government can require the use of particular enhancement technologies as a condition for individuals or organizations to engage in otherwise optional activities; for example, vaccinations can be required for foreign travel by U.S. citizens in areas where particular health threats are especially severe. These requirements can also be imposed for required, not just optional, activities; for example, most states require that parents have their children vaccinated for a variety of diseases before the children enter school. These requirements are in part for the benefit of the children who are vaccinated, as well as for "herd immunity" to protect unvaccinated children and persons with whom unvaccinated and infectious children might come into contact. Further out still on the positive end of this continuum are specific legal requirements for the use of certain enhancement technologies, with civil or possibly even criminal penalties for not doing so; there are not many instances of this kind, but examples include basic education for children and perhaps enhancement technologies aimed at reducing certain public health threats.

This same continuum covers a variety of possible negative governmental responses to enhancement technologies. An appropriate responsibility of government can be to ensure that those who make use of enhancement technologies are well informed about the potential benefits and risks of doing so. Educational programs to increase the public's understanding of the risks and benefits of the technologies need not be intended or seen as a negative policy response to the enhancement technologies in question. However, similar efforts to emphasize the risks of particular enhancement technologies may become persuasive efforts to discourage their use. Government can also provide financial or other disincentives for the use of particular enhancement technologies, for example, by taxing or regulating them heavily. Stronger negative responses include prohibitions of the use of particular enhancement technologies by persons engaged in either optional or required activities; for example, government or professional associations can ban the use of certain enhancement technologies, such as steroids for building muscle mass and strength, by individuals who participate in amateur or professional athletic activities. Finally, civil or criminal penalties can be attached to providing or using specific enhancement technologies; for example, health care professionals could face penalties for making steroids available to athletes, or for making psychopharmacological enhancement technologies with particularly unfavorable risk-benefit ratios available to children or adults.

Many governmental actions concerning enhancement technologies could be designed, not to promote or discourage their use, but to ensure that they meet standards of safety and efficacy. This possibility extends to enhancements regulations comparable to those of the Food and Drug Administration and other government bodies of medical interventions, drugs, and devices. Government regulation is used in a variety of contexts in which there is reason to believe that market forces will be inadequate to protect the public from serious risks of harm. The moral importance of individual self-determination and freedom in pursuit of one's own conception of a good life, however, supports a presumption for government neutrality toward enhancement technologies, perhaps combined with regulations for safety and efficacy. However, this presumption can be overcome by a variety of considerations that I shall pursue below.

## Who Is Using Enhancement Technologies

It is often morally important to know who is using particular enhancement technologies. I believe the most important differences are between three cases: first, when government employs the technologies, or strongly encourages or requires their use; second, when individuals decide to use the technologies for others, in particular when parents use them for their children; and, third, when individuals themselves use technologies to enhance their own capacities. One obvious important moral difference between these cases is that only the first two raise the important issue of the authority, moral or legal, of one individual, group, or institution acting in a way that can profoundly affect the life and capacities of another. A second difference, less obvious but no less important, is that different degrees and forms of neutrality are properly expected from the state, from parents acting to affect their children, and from individuals acting to affect themselves.

Let me begin with the issue of neutrality between different conceptions of a good life. An important feature of liberal political theory is that the state should seek to be neutral between different "thick" or comprehensive conceptions of a good life that its citizens may hold.[1] Liberals seek to avoid or limit the state's strongly favoring particular conceptions of a good life that not all of its citizens share. Instead, the state's role is to set the terms, or provide the institutional setting, in which all individuals can freely pursue their own different and sometimes conflicting conceptions of a good life. This liberal neutrality places substantial limits on governmental action to employ, encourage, or require the use of specific enhancement technologies that are only beneficial in some specific conceptions of a good life. The enhancements compatible with this liberal state neutrality are roughly those that fit what John Rawls called "primary goods," that is, general purpose means useful in at least a wide array of, if not virtually all, plans of life.[2] When particular enhancements have this general purpose usefulness, the state's claim that they benefit the individuals affected requires no appeal to a particular conception of a good life that those individuals may not share.

What are examples of enhancements with this general purpose usefulness? Most communities in the United States now place fluoride in the water supply to enhance individuals' normal resistance to tooth decay. Tooth decay is unwanted and harmful from virtually any perspective or conception of a good life, and so the state may legitimately take steps to enhance individuals' capacities to avoid it without violating any commitment to liberal neutrality. Government also requires for roughly the same reasons that parents send their children to school up to age 16. Education can be, I believe, properly understood as an enhancement technology, taking "technology" in a broad sense, because it is aimed at enhancing a wide array of cognitive and other capacities. Basic education does not fit a person for only a few life plans or conceptions of a good life, but is necessary, or at least useful, in a very broad array of life plans within modern societies. Consequently, requiring basic education for all children does not violate liberal state neutrality. Of course, disagreement about whether the state can legitimately employ enhancement technologies with more limited usefulness may reflect deeper disagreements within political philosophy about the extent to which the state either can or should attempt to remain neutral between different conceptions of a good life. This disagreement is a fundamental issue dividing liberal and communitarian political philosophers.

I turn now to the case of individuals using technologies to enhance the capacities of other persons; parents' use of such technologies to enhance their children's capacities is the paradigm example. Whoever has primary responsibility for raising children—in most societies, their parents—must have significant discretion in the values they impart, as well as in the particular capacities that they seek to develop and enhance in their children.[3] The degree of neutrality between different conceptions of a good life that liberal political theory asks of the state is neither possible nor desirable from parents raising their own children. Parents should have significant discretion in the use of enhancement technologies for their children, based both on the values they want to transmit to their children and on their assessment of their children's capabilities and interests; for example, whether to provide music lessons or sports camps or computer courses. The alternatives available to parents may come to include psychopharmacologic or genetic engineering, although these prospects are mostly still in the future and not well defined.

There are moral limits, however, on the authority of parents to enhance their children's capacities, as the following case illustrates. Suppose parents put their nine-year-old child into an intensive tennis training program aimed at developing the child's capacities to become a professional tennis player. This enhancement program aims at a very specific plan of life for the child and also attempts to bring the child to share the goals and plans the parents have for it. It is generally accepted that parents have a right to put their children into such programs even if others may doubt the wisdom of their doing so. But suppose the parents also said that the child's education was interfering with attempts to develop her capacity as a tennis player, and so proposed to remove her from school. Public policy, quite properly, would not permit them to do so.

This child's parents have selected a very specific plan of life for her, and now propose to enhance her capacity for that life at the cost of severely limiting or neglecting many other capacities and opportunities she would otherwise have to choose among many other different plans of life. One way of characterizing why the parents' plan for their child is wrong is that it would violate what Joel Feinberg has called a child's right to an open future.[4] Parents do not have an unlimited moral right to shape their children, and their children's capacities, at the cost of denying them a reasonable array of opportunities to select and pursue their own conception of a good life as they mature and develop the capacities to make those choices. A child needs at least a basic education to ensure those opportunities. Children's right to an open future is derivative from the more fundamental moral right of adults to self-determination in making significant decisions about their own lives for themselves and according to their own values or conception of a good life. Disagreements will arise, of course, about the extent or scope of a child's right to an open future, and about what actions would violate that right, but the right places significant limits on the use of enhancement technologies by parents for their children. In other cases, this same right can support parents' use of enhancement technologies that have the effect of enlarging and strengthening their children's capacities and opportunities to choose and effectively pursue a wide range of life choices. Basic education has this effect, and in the future some psycho-pharmacologic or genetic engineering technique, for example, increased general memory capacities, could have the same effect.

When individuals use enhancement technologies for themselves, that is, to enhance their own capacities, no neutrality between different conceptions of a good life is called for, neither the strong neutrality required of the liberal state, nor the much more limited neutrality required of parents with their children. An individual's choices—of a specific plan of life, and to enhance the capacities necessary for that plan of life—are exercises of self-determination, not impingements on another's self-determination. Public policy may legitimately seek to ensure that such choices are well informed, particularly when they carry significant and irreversible risks; but as long as individuals have normal decision-making capacities, they have a right to make such choices, even when they do so foolishly and with consequences that they may later come to regret. It may be wise for individuals to develop and enhance their capacities in ways that don't unduly close off future opportunities, including opportunities to revise and change their plan of life, but it is neither the responsibility nor the right of others, either the state or other individuals, to ensure they do so.

I have explored the issue of the appropriate neutrality regarding different conceptions of a good life expected of the state, of parents toward their children, and of individuals when their actions principally affect themselves, to illustrate why who is employing a particular en-hancement technology is important to the legitimacy of their doing so. There are other reasons why who is using an human enhancement technology is important. It is widely accepted that individuals are entitled to take risks for themselves that they would not be justified in imposing on or choosing for others. For example, individuals can volunteer to undergo high-risk medical procedures in therapeutic or research contexts, for which they would not be permitted to volunteer another for whom they are responsible. When enhancement technologies like psychopharmacologic or genetic engineering carry significant risks, for example, from uncertainty about their more subtle or long-term effects, they may be acceptable for individuals to use themselves, but not to use for others such as their children. While there is not space here to pursue this issue further, I believe there are additional respects, besides the appropriate neutrality regarding conceptions of a good life and the appropriate levels of risk that can be assumed, which make who would use an enhancement technology important for the overall assessment of whether that use is morally justified.

## Enhancements and the Concept of Benefit

One source of concern about whether public policy should promote enhancements may be linked to whether particular enhancements would in fact produce a benefit.[5] There are several reasons why the benefits of enhancements may seem more problematic than those of treatments. First, some putative enhancements might be beneficial not for the individual who undergoes the change, but only for others. For example, in Aldous Huxley's *Brave New World* the class of persons called "Deltas" were engineered to be satisfied with boring and relatively menial work.[6] This engineering was thought to benefit the larger society by providing persons willing and only able to take and fill these social roles. It was not a genuine enhancement, however, since there was no pretense that it was good for the Deltas to be created with these limited capacities. Second, some paternalistic enhancements allow others to believe that a person has benefited by undergoing a change, though the individual him or herself does not believe the change to be beneficial. In Peter Kramer's book, *Listening to Prozac*, he describes a patient on Prozac who lost his bristly and curmudgeonly qualities and became less dissatisfied and critical.[7] Although others may have preferred his new persona, he felt he had lost a central part of the character that had defined him.

Setting aside these two kinds of cases as not genuine enhancements, can we say that what is a disease, and so what counts as a treatment of disease, is objective in a way that what counts as an enhancement is not? For example, loss of sight or mobility seems to be objectively and uncontroversially bad for a person, and any treatment of a disease which prevents such losses would likewise be objectively and uncontroversially a benefit. Contrast them with enhancing the capacity to play a musical instrument or to excel in athletics. Some people have no desire to play music or athletics, and would see neither enhancement as a benefit. Similarly, from some radical positions in the disability rights movement, even the loss of hearing is not a harm. We can, however, set aside that kind of radical challenge; a sense capacity like hearing is plausibly considered a general purpose means, useful and important in nearly any life plan, although that is not to say that individuals cannot accommodate their life plans to its loss. Musical skill or excellence in athletics, by contrast, are only benefits within some, but not all, life plans.

This assertion is not, however, a general contrast between harms prevented by the treatment of disease and benefits from enhancements. First, some impairments from disease are only harms within particular life plans; for example, certain fine motor skills are needed by a pianist but are not called on in most other life plans. Second, there are potential enhancements of general purpose means, such as memory or the capacity to focus one's attention, that would be beneficial within virtually any life plan. Thus, there is no systematic difference between the benefits from enhancements and the harms prevented by the treatment of disease that makes the latter objective in a way the former are not. There are enhancements that would be a benefit within nearly any life plan, others that would be a benefit in most but not all life plans, and still others that would be a benefit only within very specific and unusual life plans. Public policy should reflect these differences and take as one goal to ensure that enhancements are used only by and for persons for whom they would in fact be a genuine benefit. Whether any particular change in an individual's conditions or capacities is a beneficial enhancement must be assessed against that individual's particular aims, plans, and values.

## Are the Means Used to Enhance Capacities Morally Important?

Besides the different ends at which enhancements aim, they also differ in the means used to achieve those ends. If we consider only the three paradigm cases of cosmetic surgery, psychopharmacology, and genetic engineering, one important difference in means emerges. Nei-

ther surgery to change physical appearance, nor a pill to change psychological traits, nor genetic intervention to change or shape an individual's
genome, involves substantial discipline and effort to produce the desired
feature or capability. For example, altering a fundamental character
trait or psychological feature by a "quick fix" of "popping a pill" seems
to some people too easy and less admirable than changing that same
trait or feature through hard-earned insight psychotherapy. One method
engages our uniquely human, rational capacities, while the other bypasses
them and works directly on our brain chemistry. The moral or policy
significance of distinctions like this one is problematic and I shall not
pursue it further, but only make a general point about the importance
of means.

Sometimes a valued human activity is defined in part by the means
it employs, not just by the end at which it aims. Consider two examples.
In some sports, building body strength and mass through physical training
is an appropriate means of enhancing those features, whereas doing so
by the use of steroids is not. Our understanding of the nature of the
sport includes not just the final performance itself, but also the means
by which the capacities for that performance are gained. Given that
understanding, the use of steroids bypasses a relevant part of the sport—
physical training—and amounts to a kind of cheating on the means that
are appropriate to achieving success in the sport. The second example
comes from chess. It was a great achievement when IBM's computer
"Big Blue" recently beat the world chess champion, Gary Kasparov. But
it surely was a very different achievement than if a human challenger
had beaten Kasparov. And suppose the IBM engineer who implemented
the moves that Big Blue chose claimed that *he* had beaten Kasparov,
albeit by unorthodox means? Here, means make all the difference in
the chess skills and successes with which the engineer should be credited.
In many valued human activities, the means of acquiring the capacities
required for the activity are as much valued and admired as the performance of the activity. They are a part of the very definition of the activity,
and transforming them transforms, and can devalue, the activity itself.

## The Importance of the Magnitude of Enhancements

Most enhancements of human capacities or traits can be distinguished
by the magnitude of changes produced. If the capacity or trait is in
general beneficial to a person, then it might be thought that the more
it is enhanced, the greater the benefit. But that would be wrong for

at least two kinds of reasons. First, some enhancements are only beneficial within a limited range because of how the enhanced capacity or trait interacts with the individual's other capacities or traits. Beyond that range, further enhancement of a particular property may interact in sufficiently undesirable ways with the individual's other properties to make the change, all things considered, a harm instead of a benefit. It is recognized, for example, that humans have different forms of memory. We can imagine enhancements of a particular form of memory that so crowds out others forms of memory and/or other cognitive processes as to be overall a harm instead of a benefit; enhancements of that form of memory within a limited range, however, are a benefit.

The second reason why some enhancements would only be beneficial within a limited range is that beyond that range individuals would become unsuited for human social life. There are social and economic advantages to being tall; that is why growth hormone that can raise a normal individual's height to several inches above the norm would be a beneficial enhancement. But there are limits to how much of an increase in height would be beneficial. To be nine feet tall would on balance be harmful in nearly any human society because our social world is constructed for persons whose height rarely reaches beyond seven feet. One would literally become, in a physical respect, unfit for human company. And if the change were still more dramatic, as in the case of Gulliver in Lilliput, then it could become hard even to see the individual as a member of the same species.[8] Many changes in human features and capacities would only be beneficial enhancements within some range, and public policy could quite appropriately regulate or otherwise limit the use of enhancement technologies to ensure that the gain stays within the beneficial range.

## A Miscellany of Other Moral Problems with Enhancements

I now want to state very briefly several miscellaneous moral problems concerning enhancements of human capacities that have significant bearing on public policy. The first problem arises when an enhancement confers a competitive or positional advantage on its recipient, thereby strengthening his or her position relative to others in competitions for scarce roles or benefits. If the enhancement is not generally available to all who might want it and benefit from it, but is expensive and distributed on the basis of ability to pay, then only the economically well-off will get it. This problem raises concerns about fairness and equality of opportunity. Specifically, individuals whose competitive position for a particular role or benefit is worsened as a result of their inability to afford the enhancement can complain that they no longer have a fair opportunity to compete for the benefit against those who have purchased the competitive enhancement. Each of the three paradigm cases of enhancements provide examples of this problem. Since being physically attractive is an advantage in work and other contexts, expensive cosmetic surgery can confer this advantage. If expensive medications like Prozac can improve an individual's self-confidence, that too can be a significant advantage in work and other contexts. And if genetic interventions someday become possible to enhance a capacity like memory, or specific forms of memory, that too would provide a competitive advantage in work and other contexts. Of course, we already tolerate the distribution of many competitive advantages, including enhancements such as higher quality private school education, largely on the basis of ability to pay, and we might tolerate distributing these new enhancements on that basis as well. But tolerating unfairness hardly makes it less unfair. If significant competitive benefits accrue from new abilities to enhance human capacities available only on an ability to pay basis, their use will raise serious issues of fairness for public policy.

The second moral problem arises when an enhancement is likely to be used by nearly everyone because it is thought to confer a significant competitive or positional advantage and is widely available—perhaps because it is funded through health insurance or other social welfare programs or because it is so inexpensive that nearly everyone can afford it. An example, although it is certainly not a low-cost intervention, is the use of growth hormone to secure the advantage that comes with increased height. If all parents used growth hormone to increase their children's height, no children would gain any relative advantage because all children's height would be increased and no one's height relative to others would change. The attempt to gain a competitive advantage from an enhancement available to everyone will be self-defeating. The case of growth hormone illustrates not only the lack of any benefit from universally available competitive enhancements, but also the waste of resources and the assumption of needless risks from use of the enhancement.

Public policy can reasonably limit the use of enhancements that would be unfair or self-defeating. But there is a complication. Many enhancements likely to become possible will in part confer competitive or positional advantages, and in part constitute intrinsic goods that confer noncompetitive benefits. Suppose, for example, that it becomes possible in the future through either psychopharmacology or genetic interventions to improve individuals' capacity to focus their attention for significant time on a particular task or activity. Many adults with no disease or deficit now use the drug Ritalin for this purpose.[9] Its use clearly confers an important competitive advantage to individuals in work contexts. But it also increases the intrinsic satisfactions those individuals obtain from activities like listening to music, watching films or sunsets, and so forth, none of which are competitive benefits. The quandary for public policy is that concerns about fairness or avoiding self-defeating interventions supports limits on the use of such enhancements, but these limits at the same time deny individuals the opportunity of gaining significant noncompetitive, intrinsic benefits.

The third moral problem for public policy concerns enhancement technologies that, at least in some contexts, hold out the possibility of significant benefits, but also appear to have problematic or clearly unfavorable risk/benefit ratios. Two relatively polar policy options exist for dealing with serious risks, which we have seen mirrored in other public policy contexts, such as regulating risks in the workplace and regulating drugs and devices. The aim of public policy can be to ensure that individuals have full information regarding the risks and benefits of an enhancement, leaving them free to determine for themselves whether the risk/benefit ratio is acceptable; this approach is the one taken, through requirements of informed consent, with most high-risk medical treatments for serious medical conditions. The alternative is a strong regulatory oversight process in which enhancements must satisfy a clearly favorable risk/benefit ratio, or be without significant risks, to be permitted. This approach more closely approximates the alternative we have taken with drugs and devices, or with hazardous conditions like carcinogens in the workplace. There are, of course, many alternative policy positions which strike different balances between leaving informed individuals free to make their own choices, on the one hand, and paternalistic regulatory protection of individuals against serious risks, on the other.

Especially for genetic and psychopharmacological enhancements, there will often be substantial uncertainty about both their benefits and risks. Some enhancements may have relatively broad effects on complex, multifactorial traits, sometimes stretching out over considerable time and resulting in considerable controversy and uncertainty about a particular enhancement's overall degree of risk and potential for benefit. If public policy seeks to regulate acceptable risks, controversy is inevitable about when the risks of a potential enhancement are too high to justify permitting it. Sufficient latitude will be needed in such enhancements to accommodate reasonable disagreements between persons about when the risk/benefit ratios are acceptable. Germline genetic enhancements, for example, carry much greater uncertainty and risks, since they have the potential to affect large numbers of persons as they are passed on across generations.

The fourth problem concerns a potential bad effect of enhancements whose precise nature and likely extent are both speculative at present. When one person employs extensive enhancements to shape the nature and capacities of another person, most typically in parent-child contexts, the parent may view the child as an object to be molded to fit the parents' aims and values, not a unique individual whose character, capacities, and life history should be permitted to unfold according to its own nature. This attitude reflects an objectification of the child by its parents and a failure to respect it as an autonomous individual, an attitude that should be discouraged, not encouraged. The second part of this concern is the potential effect on the individual who is the subject of the objectification. If one has been extensively shaped by another person, one might lose one's sense of self-creation and individuality, both of which depend on the belief that one has significant capacity to control and determine over time the kind of person one becomes by the choices and commitments one makes. If many traits essential to individuals' sense of their own identity now have to be understood as having been specifically selected for them by others, then they become not the deliberate creations of their own doing and choices, but products of the doings and choices of others. The concern is that individuals may come to see themselves more like objects that have been manipulated by others than like agents who have created themselves. This concern was strongly expressed by many opponents of human cloning in the wake of the cloning of a sheep, and it applies in a more limited form to enhancements of human beings.

The fifth problem with enhancement technologies concerns those that create competitive or positional advantages for some individuals, but at the cost of significant adverse consequences for others. When some individuals use enhancement technologies to gain competitive advantages for themselves, they put coercive pressure on others to use them as well so as to avoid becoming worse off than they were initially. One of the most familiar examples is the use of steroids in high school and college athletics. When some athletes use steroids to gain physical bulk and strength, others with whom they compete will be strongly pressured to use them as well, even if they would prefer not to assume the risks of doing so. Failing to use the steroids may effectively bar them from athletic participation or success. The task for public policy is to determine when the frequency and seriousness of coercive pressures to use risky or expensive enhancement technologies are sufficient to warrant prohibition or regulation of the use of the technologies; for example, public policy now generally restricts the use of steroids in high school athletics, but permits the use of expensive specialized courses for high school students to improve their scores on SAT tests.

Finally, would some individuals' use of enhancement technologies create additional harms to other persons, besides a worsened competitive position and coercive pressures to use the enhancement themselves? Any full answer to this question will require experience with the nature of the enhancements that become possible and the indirect effects they have on others, but there is one kind of potential harm that it is worth signaling at this time. Consider the prevention of disabilities that disability rights advocates have claimed is harmful to other persons with the disabilities.[10] For example, testing is typically recommended for pregnant women over age thirty-five for the genetically transmitted disorder of Down's syndrome. Women who find that their fetus has this disorder typically abort the fetus and try again for a normal pregnancy. Disability rights advocates have argued that this practice harms persons who have Down's syndrome by sending a message that their lives are not worth living, and that it would have been better if they had never been born. They argue that these judgments are implicit in any woman's deliberate decision to abort a fetus with Down's syndrome to prevent it from coming into existence, and that they demean and devalue the lives of persons with Down's syndrome. Defenders of the testing respond that no message is sent that persons with Down's syndrome don't have lives worth living, nor that they should be killed, but only that if it is possible to create a person without this disability instead of a person with it, it is reasonable to prefer the former.

This issue is complex and unresolved, though my own view is that the charge of the disability rights proponent can be met. But the point here is that enhancements may raise issues similar to the disabilities case. Indeed, in one respect the implicit message of some enhancements may be worse because they may respond only to prejudicial stereotypes about some groups, not real differences in function produced by disabilities like Down's syndrome. For example, suppose a person has a "hooked nose" of a sort stereotypically associated with Jewish persons, and seeks cosmetic surgery to rid herself of this feature of her appearance. As in the disabilities case, it could be argued that this "enhancement" sends a message to other Jews that it is better not to have this supposed mark of being Jewish, and that being Jewish is somehow to be inferior. Cosmetic surgery in a case like this reinforces stereotypes and prejudices about Jews, and is thereby harmful to other Jews. Similar cases may arise in the future with genetic engineering. Suppose it became possible to change a person's genes for skin color, and some African-American parents sought a genetic intervention to change the color of their future children's skin from black to white. Here again, their action would clearly send a message that they considered it to be a burden to have black skin, and would play into deeply harmful prejudices and stereo-types about African-Americans. African-Americans could argue that the values this "enhancement" expresses are harmful to them by reinforcing the prejudices and stereotypes of white society about them. These two cases illustrate that it is a mistake to think that the only harm some people's enhancements could cause to others is to put them at a competi-tive disadvantage. Serious harms can come to others from the value judgments that enhancements express that devalue and degrade them.

## Who Should Pay for the Enhancement Technology?

The final public policy issue that I will take up here is whether human enhancement technologies, particularly those employed in medi-cal contexts or using what we intuitively think of as medical means, should be covered and funded by health insurance, such as private health insurance or public health insurance programs like Medicare and Medicaid, or by other social welfare programs. Here is one argument that enhancements should not be covered by health insurance. The aim of medicine is commonly agreed to be the promotion and protection of health; health is the absence of disease, therefore, medicine's aim should be the treatment or prevention of disease. Enhancement of normal function is neither the prevention nor treatment of disease; therefore, enhancement of human function is not properly part of medicine. The proper role of health insurance is to protect and promote health by funding medical care. This argument vastly oversimplifies some very complex and controversial issues, but if something like it is correct, then only the treatment or prevention of disease, not the enhancement of normal function, should be covered by health insurance. However, this apparently straightforward argument for excluding enhancement technologies from coverage by health insurance is problematic for several reasons.

First, some services that are properly and standardly covered by health insurance do not treat or prevent disease; for example, abortion services are typically covered by health insurance, but a normal pregnancy is not a disease and its termination by an abortion is not medical treatment, although it is typically done by medical personnel using medical means. There can be sound public policy reasons for funding certain services under health insurance, although those services do not treat or prevent disease.

Second, every service that does treat or prevent disease need not be covered by health insurance. Some treatments are excluded from coverage because they are experimental, although they are clearly intended as treatment. Moreover, some nonexperimental treatments may not be covered by health insurance because of reasonable resource limits under which health insurance plans operate. Fair procedures to allocate scarce resources can reasonably exclude some low-benefit/high-cost medical treatments. An account of the just allocation of resources to and within health care, not simply a determination of what is medical treatment for a disease, is necessary to determine which treatments should be covered under health insurance. Moreover, as we will see shortly, the reasons that a theory of justice requires the funding of most treatments in public or private health insurance programs might warrant the funding of some enhancements as well.

Finally, some enhancements are intended to prevent disease, and so should be covered and funded according to the standard rationale for health insurance as covering services for the treatment and prevention of disease. Perhaps the most straightforward example is vaccination programs. Vaccinations for specific diseases enhance the normal immune system's ability to respond to and prevent those diseases. More general enhancements of the body's capacity to respond to and prevent a broad array of diseases may become possible through genetic interventions. In either case, these medical enhancements are for the prevention of disease and therefore should be eligible for coverage by health insurance like other preventive interventions. Thus, there are several respects in which the treatment/enhancement distinction does not mark the line between services that should be covered and services that should be excluded from coverage in private or public health insurance plans.

## Does Equality of Opportunity Support Limiting Health Insurance Coverage to Treatment, but Not Enhancement?

The conclusion stated at the end of the preceding section can be reinforced by delving in more depth into the reason why it is widely agreed that access to medical treatment should be guaranteed to all citizens by public or private health insurance. In the most well-developed and widely accepted theory of justice in health care, Norman Daniels argues that the provision of health care is a matter of justice because of its role in maintaining or restoring normal function, which in turn helps maintain fair equality of opportunity for all citizens.[11] Fair equality of opportunity is the fundamental moral principle underlying the typical restriction of health insurance coverage to the treatment or prevention of disease. Could enhancements of normal human function also promote fair equality of opportunity? They could if the same disadvantage can be present in an individual who is at the low end of normal function, but has no disease that requires treatment, as in a person whose disadvantage is caused by disease that can be treated. Our concern for equality would then extend beyond eliminating inequalities of opportunity caused by disease to inequalities whose removal would count as enhancement, not treatment.

The problem for grounding claims to treatment, but not enhancement, in equality of opportunity is understanding why the same disadvantage should have a claim on social resources for its removal when it is caused by disease, but not when it is within the range of normal human function and in the absence of disease. David Allen and Norman Fost's case of two children who are both of predicted short stature illustrates the problem.[12] The first child, Johnny, has a deficiency in the production of growth hormone as a result of a brain tumor that has been successfully treated; his predicted adult height is five feet three inches, significantly below the norm for adult males in his society. The second child, Billy, secretes normal levels of growth hormone, but has short parents; he too has an expected adult height of five feet three inches. Short stature is a social and economic disadvantage in our society; each boy suffers from this same undeserved disadvantage. Only Johnny, however, has a disease that impairs function, that is, his deficient production of growth hormone, whose treatment would result in an expected increase in his adult stature. But there is good reason to believe that giving growth hormone to Billy, whose production of it is already in the normal range, would produce the same increase in his expected adult height as for

Johnny. Thus, if we want to rectify undeserved disadvantages in order to secure fair equality of opportunity, why should only Johnny, but not Billy, receive growth hormone?

Concern for equality and rectifying undeserved disadvantages apparently supports giving growth hormone to Billy, who has genes that will produce short stature, as much as to Johnny, who has a disease that will result in short stature. There is much more to be said about how an account of just health care grounded in a principle of fair equality of opportunity should apply to cases like this. Despite difficult cases like that of growth hormone, pragmatic concerns together with moral and political concerns that cannot be explored further here, may support use of the treatment/enhancement distinction as a rough guide to the health care that all should have as a matter of justice. The case of growth hormone does show, however, that there is no straightforward and unproblematic limiting the fair equality of opportunity account of just health care to disease only, and not to enhancements that would rectify disadvantages in opportunity caused by normal genes.

## Equality of What?

Even if fair equality of opportunity requires only access to treatment and not enhancement, a more general egalitarian concern reaches more broadly. Fair equality of opportunity would be secured, at least in health care, when no treatable disease causes an impairment of normal function and in turn of opportunity. However, remaining significant differences in people's talents and abilities would result in inequalities in opportunities and welfare. Many of these inequalities would be caused by genetic differences between persons, all of which remain within the norm for the species. Amartya Sen has argued that the proper egalitarian concern is with individuals' capabilities, or capability sets, not with fair equality of opportunity as it is typically understood by Rawls and others.[13] Individuals with significantly different levels of natural talents and abilities do not have equal capabilities to achieve satisfying and worthwhile lives. A broad egalitarian focus on capabilities has the advantage that it seeks to eliminate these genetically inherited, undeserved and unchosen inequalities between persons that the fair equality of opportunity account would leave in place.

As our knowledge of psychopharmacology and human genetics continues its exponential growth in coming years, we can expect to learn both how genes are linked to particular inequalities in capabilities and in turn how genetic or psychopharmacological interventions can reduce or eliminate many of these inequalities. For example, the range of normal memory in humans is relatively broad, and people's memory has a significant impact on their performance in a variety of social tasks and roles that in turn impact their expectations and opportunities. Interventions to enhance the memory of people at the low end of the normal range could reduce the disadvantages in capabilities they suffer.

As the important and lively "equality of what" debate over the last two decades displays, egalitarian concerns can have other alternative focuses besides fair equality of opportunity or capabilities, none of which can be pursued further here.[14] The important point for present purposes, however, is that even if treatment but not enhancement supports the protection or restoration of fair equality of opportunity, this fact does not settle whether any enhancements should be covered by health insurance or other social welfare programs. The deeper issue is what are the proper focuses of attempts to achieve equality between persons, and whether any of them are forwarded by enhancements of human functions.

## Conclusion

I shall not try in conclusion to summarize all the different respects in which I have argued human enhancement technologies may vary in ways important for public policy. The many and complex important properties of different enhancement technologies, the complex and different possible policy responses to enhancement technologies, and the different kinds of moral reasons and values that bear on them, all suggest that any policy guidelines for responding to new technologies to enhance human capacities must be highly complex and nuanced in order to take account of complexities like those I have explored in this paper.

## NOTES

1. John Rawls, *A Theory of Justice* (Cambridge, Mass.: Harvard University Press, 1971).
2. Rawls, *A Theory of Justice,* p. 90–95.
3. Ferdinand Schoeman, "Parental Discretion and Children's Rights: Background and Implications for Medical Decision-Making," *Journal of Medicine and Philosophy* 10 (1985): 45–62.

**4.** Joel Feinberg, "The Child's Right to an Open Future," in *Whose Child: Children's Rights, Parental Authority, and State Power*, ed. William Aiken and Hugh LaFollette (Totowa, N.J.: Lowman & Littlefield, 1980).

**5.** The discussion in this section draws on my work in "Why Not the Best?" Chapter 6 in Allen Buchanan, Dan W. Brock, Norman Daniels, and Daniel Wikler, *Genes and the Just Society: Genetic Intervention in the Shadow of Eugenics*, forthcoming.

**6.** Aldous Huxley, *Brave New World* (London: Chalto and Winders, 1932).

**7.** Peter Kramer, *Listening to Prozac* (New York: Viking Press, 1993).

**8.** Jonathan Swift, *Gulliver's Travels* (New York: C.I. Potter, 1980).

**9.** Lawrence H. Diller, "The Run on Ritalin: Attention Deficit Disorder and Stimulant Treatment in the 1990's," *Hastings Center Report* 26, No. 2 (1996): 12–18.

**10.** Adrienne Asch, "Can Aborting 'Imperfect' Children Be Immoral?" in *Ethical Issues in Modern Medicine,* 3rd Ed., ed. John D. Arras and Nancy K. Rhoden (Mountain View, Calif.: 1995), pp. 317–21; and Arno G. Motulsky and Jeffrey Murray, "Will Prenatal Diagnosis with Selective Abortion Affect Society's Attitude Toward the Handicapped?" in *Research Ethics* (New York: Alan R. Liss, Inc., 1983), pp. 277–91.

**11.** Norman Daniels, *Just Health Care* (New York: Cambridge University Press, 1985).

**12.** David B. Allen and Norman C. Fost, "Growth Hormone Therapy for Short Stature: Panacea or Pandora's Box?" *Journal of Pediatrics* 117 (1990): 16–21.

**13.** Amartya Sen, *Inequality Reexamined* (Cambridge, Mass.: Harvard University Press, 1992).

**14.** Norman Daniels, "Equality of What: Welfare, Resources, or Capabilities?" *Philosophy and Phenomenological Research* vol. 1, Supplement, Fall (1990): 273–96.

DAVID M. FRANKFORD

# The Treatment/Enhancement
# Distinction as an Armament
# in the Policy Wars

As children of the Enlightenment, we western moderns like to think that well-laid plans, formulated in our minds and in our deliberations, can be translated into social action without significant transformation. This manner of thinking extends to "policy," which is traditionally conceived of as a rational plan of action, deduced from justified first principles, which need only be carried out. While this aspiration for policy may be worthy, nothing of the sort occurs in the social world. Instead, the converse often obtains, for social action frequently uses "policy" as a normative and cognitive resource to justify actions taken. At the very least, the interaction is recursive, with the result that action cannot be characterized as the epiphenomenal consequence of thought.

In this Hastings Center Project we were considering whether to issue a report to policymakers to aid them in their formulation of public policy to govern enhancements to human capacity. Such a policy guideline would identify various factors relevant to the creation of such public policy and would connect those factors with appropriate policy responses. In this paper I describe what uses would likely be made of such a policy statement. While prediction is always a hazardous vocation, in this context I believe that my predictions are warranted by our experiences with somewhat analogous distinctions drawn and used for purposes of resource allocation in our current health care system.

My paper proceeds in four steps. First, I characterize the bestowal of the terms "treatment" and "enhancement" as statements of what exists and as normative conclusions rather than immanent characteristics. Here, to demonstrate that we must look at the manner in which actors in our current context use and generate "policy," I contrast Eric Juengst's sensitive discussion of the manner in which we use the terms "treatment" and "enhancement"[1] with Dan Brock's equally sensitive discussion of the policy responses that might be evoked from different forms of enhancement.[2] Second, I describe the creation of "policy" as a social process in which actors grab fragments of "policy statements" from a "field" or "library" of available policy statements and use them in their own contexts to justify their own actions, with the result that the coherence and normative foundations of such statements are transformed, lost, or even subverted. Third, I offer a contemporaneous example by discussing the manner in which our governmental and private insurance agencies are drawing a distinction between technologies that are "experimental" and those that are not, reimbursing the latter but not the former. Fourth, I contrast this administration of the treatment/enhancement distinction with the manner in which the distinction might be administered within the clinical encounter.

### The Treatment/Enhancement Distinction as an Empirical Statement and a Normative Conclusion

"That's merely an enhancement, not something that's necessary."

In his paper Eric Juengst studies the manner in which we use the terms "treatment" and "enhancement."[3] He delineates three spheres, which, although he does not explicitly say so, would appear to interact to some degree. In the first sphere, we use the treatment/enhancement distinction to delimit the nature of professional obligation. "Treatments" are interventions that professionals are obligated to perform; "enhancements" are activities that are not required but are either permissible or forbidden. Professionals might be obligated to prescribe Cognex in the treatment of Alzheimer's, for example, but merely permitted or even precluded from its use to increase a child's SAT scores. By contrast, in the second sphere we use the terms to debate whether an intervention is appropriate in the context of a particular life activity. Continuing the previous example, one might claim that chessplayers should be banned from using Cognex to enhance their play. Finally, in the third sphere, we use the treatment/enhancement distinction to differentiate interventions that are "needed" from those that are merely "preferred," funding the latter with shared resources but the former from personal ones alone. To finish the example, then, the use of Cognex as a treatment for Alzheimer's will be a service covered by health care insurance, while its use to compete for higher SAT scores or in chess will not.

Two points are particularly noteworthy. First, in each sphere the uses of the terms are permeable. In each we draw upon a set of distinctions to justify a particular ontological statement and normative conclusion. It would be argued, then, that the use of Cognex to treat memory "loss" in Alzheimer's "restores" a "natural" function, one founded in biological processes, and an attribute of species-typical functioning. By contrast, using Cognex to play chess better creates "additional" memory, akin to that of a computer, and hence something that is "artificial," like the computer's "memory," founded in technology not biology and not an element of species-typical functioning. However, as Juengst suggests, each of these categories, too, is permeable, as mind shades into body, and the natural into the social.

Second, in each sphere the terms are derivative. When we use the terms to delimit professional obligation, we draw on our sense regarding the limits of professional knowledge, the ethical implications of those limits, and the manner in which our "humanity" exceeds the boundaries those limits imply. The use of Cognex for Alzheimer's, then, is medically appropriate and indicated because an appropriate use of pharmacology is to restore the inability to remember one's identity, where one lives, and one's relatives. This use is directed at the end of personal and familial suffering. By contrast, when we use the terms to discuss personal obligation, we draw on our sense of the nature of the activity to be affected. Thus, when we conclude that the use of Cognex to play chess is an enhancement, we call upon the characteristic of the activity we call chess, the norms of competition used in the game, and the manner in which the activity would or would not be destroyed by the use of Cognex. Finally, when we decide whether Cognex should be covered as a treatment, we discuss such matters as how much it would cost in various uses, whether that cost can be afforded, and how it would be fairly distributed.

When these two points are combined, we can understand that calling a particular use of an intervention a "treatment" or an "enhancement" is an ontological statement and a normative conclusion. Given the permeability of the distinction, nothing immanent in a particular technology or its biological effect determines that the technology is inexorably a treatment or enhancement. Further, given that the normative conclusion follows from such considerations as we have here discussed, the treatment/enhancement distinction is not a foundation for moral justification but the result of justification itself. That is not to conclude, of course, that the terms are somehow useless. They are part of our vocabulary concerning what is and what ought to be, and, as such, we share an intersubjective use. Yet what this implies is that we must pay attention to the social processes by which the labels "treatment" and "enhancement" would be applied to particular interventions.

It is the lack of this discussion in Dan Brock's paper that troubles me.[4] In a sense, Brock's paper follows naturally from Juengst's because Brock perceptively teases out the policy implications that might follow from the conclusion that an intervention is an enhancement. Policymakers may thus require that certain enhancements be performed, variously encourage the performance of others, and prohibit the use of others still. Such disparate policy treatments might follow from consideration of who is using the enhancement, with due attention to the moral limits on different spheres of authority. Decisions affecting such questions as who will pay for enhancements and who will obtain the benefit of such payments would have recourse to some theory of distributive justice.

The difficulty I wish to pinpoint here is that the neat cleavage between the papers is misleading. If I am correct that the treatment/enhancement distinction is an ontological statement and a normative conclusion rather than a premise, then one of the subjects of public policy will be the decision whether to label an intervention as an enhancement to begin with, something that Brock seems to take as a premise. Moreover, the decision whether so to label an intervention will recursively take into account the social consequences of such a naming. Consequently, to the extent that public policy stipulates the manner in which enhancements are treated, that policy reflects back on the manner in which the treatment/enhancement distinction itself is then drawn. Thus, again: to decide whether to issue a policy product and to determine its content, one must consider the social processes in which this treatment/enhancement distinction will be employed.

## Rules, Regulations, and Privileges in the Policy Library

Organizational theorists have long noticed that actual practices in organizations are decoupled from formal policy statements.[5] Similarly, students of public policy have long known that policy is rarely implemented as formulated.[6] These observations are not simply the result of the fact that consequences can never be fully anticipated or that word is often separated from deed.[7] Rather, the "problem" relates to the very stuff of policy. Policy is not the rational connection of ends to means, the properly calibrated choice of inducements, rules, rights, and penalties, but rather consists in the rhetorical making of a case—the statement of what is and what ought to be—by the use of such tropes as stories, synecdoche, metaphor, and ambiguity.[8]

My description of policy starts with language because one must break in somewhere, and because this particular starting point seems defensible, given that our social world and language are one and the same,[9] and that the ontological status of any other starting point is itself dependent on language.[10] Our language tells us that society is organized into what might be called "action-units"—individuals, associations, organizations, the state—which our language "creates" as entities and as agents endowed with, first, purposes; second, means; third, rationality, which for present purposes I shall discuss as means-end rationality; and fourth, action.[11] Going in the opposite direction, our language describes actors who take actions, which are the consequence of the actor's formulation of a purpose, a canvassing of the means to achieve that future state of affairs, and the ability to calculate rationally the appropriate means to be used to attain those ends.[12]

Actors, however, do not "exist" in isolation; rather, our language "situates" them in a field of constraint and opportunity. Hence only certain moves in the field are endowed with legitimacy,[13] and moves bring certain repercussions, which constrain action further,[14] but likewise open up new possibilities.[15] To reiterate, because the definitions of actions are both creations and creatures of language, this field is likewise linguistic; society is text.[16]

"Policy" comprises an important part of this text. Policy consists of statements of what exists and what ought to be. More specifically, policy statements constitute needs, interests, and causes; and, by defining the rational, good, and right, policy statements also formulate legitimate ends, means appropriate to attain those ends, and standards governing the connection between means and ends.

This field of policy, however, should not be taken as static; nor should it be taken as unitary or completely separate from actors. Rather, at any time diverse and possibly inconsistent policy statements are available to constitute an actor's policy.[17] Following Foucault, the field of available policy statements may be thought of as a "library."[18] Policy is successfully formulated when its discourse links together and imposes a coherence on statements located in and borrowed from this library.[19] Yet analysis of such policy need not take this coherence to be the essential nature of policy but must instead problematize it to describe the manner in which that coherence is imposed. Put differently and ironically, to grasp the coherence of policy we must understand an incoherent process.

This process is quite strategic.[20] In the policy wars of political and social struggle certain statements of policy may be enunciated. These conditions of possibility and constraint are internal to the rules of the policy language game, which stipulates what policy consists in, whether its formulation may be described as "voluntary" or "determined," and, if a particular agent may be given credit for it, who that agent may be. The game is always in progress, and thus in a given present the game plays itself by constituting some policy statements as universals, the eternal *logos* that has always been, has a ubiquitous present, and will always be. These policy statements, analogous to the scientific facts described by Latour,[21] are powerful because they have been separated from their context of articulation, and thereby made "devoid of any trace of ownership, construction, time and place. [They] could have been known for centuries or handed down by God Himself together with the Ten Commandments."[22] Other policy statements are weak because they have been characterized as contextual and thereby contingent. With regard to these statements, the game plays itself by constituting actors, who—it is said—adopt, modify, or reject other (universal) statements of policy because of their particular interests alone. "Their" statements are discredited by guilt of association.

The crucial plays of the game, therefore, consist in the manner in which statements become linked into chains, forming "policy networks."[23] Sometimes these linkages are virtually impregnable by virtue of the fact that one policy statement becomes incorporated in another policy statement, which in turn is embedded in another, in a seemingly endless discursive chain. These statements recognize and reinforce each other's coherence. Together they stand, fight, and attempt to disperse themselves—conquer other statements—as a tightly woven and seamless discursive formation, which constitutes technically feasible and legitimate action—"goals," "problems," and "solutions."[24] Other times the connection between statements is open to challenge. Their claim that together they form a coherent whole that must be imposed on other statements is successfully parried, as by the assertion that another policy statement is context-bound—designed for circumstances or values quite different from "ours" such that "our" policy must not link up with "theirs."[25] In "this" situation, there is greater freedom of action because those "other" statements have authority only in that "other" context but no authority "here." This process of binding and unbinding, inclusion and exclusion, freedom and constraint, creates stable yet fluid policy networks, and the process of formulating policy thus may be termed "structured chaos," "chaotic structure," or even "organized anarchy."[26] Further, this process is recursive: as a discursive formation of policy statements is constituted, defended, and imposed as coherent, that formation reorders the library, shaping the collection and the lending privileges for other policy statements, delimiting the linkages that may be formed among them, and yet also opening up new strategies.

Hence, the impact of any policy statement is going to depend upon the manner in which it relates to other policy statements and the strength of that combination as a mode of justification.[27] A powerful policy statement will impose the coherence of its linkages on other actors' statements. It will become part of a relatively unassailable policy network, and any actor's discourse that attempts to ignore it or act contrary to its "command" will do so at its peril. By contrast, a policy statement that is weak will be ignored, or reduced to a fragment and torn from its moorings in that it will be incorporated in a justificatory framework wholly at odds with that in which it was first or previously articulated. This weak statement will be severed from the discursive linkages it wishes to impose and will instead be forced into unforeseen, unpredictable, or undesirable alliances with other statements.

Our question, therefore, concerns the strength of a Hastings Center Project's policy statement that would draw a treatment/enhancement distinction around a theory of justice.[28] Would that coherence impose itself on others' statements? For better or worse, my prediction is that such a statement would be reduced to a fragment.

To begin, a statement that formulates a treatment/enhancement distinction potentially makes that distinction "real." More than likely, current political and social discourse concerning health care policy would validate the "reality" of such a distinction because, as the previous section discusses, that ontology meshes very well with our language of professional obligation, personal agency, and questions of distribution. However, the rules that allow and enable the enunciation of this reality would not necessarily force other agents to link it with the statements that our policy statement would say are necessary associates, to wit, statements concerning distributive justice. I believe that this "norm" of dissociation would follow from three aspects of our current discursive formation. First, in our current context policies formulated around considerations of distributive justice are just not playing very well, particularly in the health care sector. We need only reflect upon the recent demise of health-insurance reform to understand that point. Second, what does play right now, again particularly in health care, are policies that stress technical efficiency,[29] and technical efficiency as a means to increase the size of the overall pie: the greatest goodies for the greatest number—utilitarianism (but nothing like sophisticated hybrid consequentialist models that attempt to account for distributive concerns).[30] Third, in order to make the pie "grow"—that is, the concern to limit health care expenditures because they disrupt economic growth—normative questions are being converted left and right into scientific questions.[31] We participants in this project may state that such conversions constitute a fundamental error—that a confusion between factual and normative modes of justification renders such practices incoherent. Unfortunately, this point seems to be lost to most health care policy. It is our criteria for coherence that are deemed to be incoherent and therefore deserving of marginalization.

In sum, I would bet at least some of the farm that our legitimation of a treatment/enhancement distinction would indeed be constitutive of reality. The distinction would then be reified in the form of public and private insurance coverage decisions, made with reference to a definition of the good, most probably utilitarianism, such that the distinction would become a tool for wrong. Also, the primary definition of good used would be rationalization, or, in other words, formalization in the service of technical efficiency. Finally, the distinction would be "naturalized" in the sense that it will be pled and accepted that some technologies are *an sich* enhancements—despite any of our protestations to the contrary—and these matters of "fact" will be turned over to scientific inquiry.

## A Contemporaneous Example: The Distinction between Experimental and Nonexperimental Treatments

An analogy may be drawn between a treatment/enhancement distinction and a distinction commonly drawn between experimental and nonexperimental treatments.[32] This analogy is apt for three reasons. First, the experimental/nonexperimental dichotomy is a part of our vocabulary to distinguish among types of biomedical interventions. This distinction is used to delineate professional obligation, particularly with regard to informed consent, and is commonly employed in both public and private health insurance to separate covered from noncovered services. Second, the experimental/nonexperimental distinction is often justified by normative argument similar to that used to distinguish treatment from enhancement.[33] Experimental interventions, it is argued, are just a frill, not reasonable and necessary for the treatment of illness, but instead merely desired as a matter of personal predilection. Put differently, until the effectiveness of an intervention has been established, no individual can successfully claim that the intervention promotes species-typical functioning. As such, the individual desiring such an intervention has no legitimate warrant on the health insurance commons, whether public or private. Further, given scarcity of resources, coverage of nonexperimental treatments squanders limited resources. In the zero-sum game of Medicaid, for example, coverage of liver transplants means that there is then less money for prenatal care, children's dental services, and the like. Third, the experimental/nonexperimental treatment distinction is often justified by prudential considerations.[34] Most significantly, it is commonly claimed that there is a strong social interest in verifying or falsifying the purported efficacy of an experimental intervention, particularly through phase III clinical trials. However, if the intervention becomes covered by insurance, it is quickly diffused, with the result that there is no longer an incentive to undertake long and expensive randomized controlled trials. "Society," the argument runs, should therefore deny coverage of an experimental intervention to force proponents of its use to spend the necessary resources for its proper evaluation.

Note initially three points about these policy arguments. First, as is true of all policy statements, they assume an ontological category because they impliedly claim that certain interventions *are* simply experimental. Put differently, they implicitly reject any notion that these categories have an element of social construction, that our policy process is involved in creating them and determining which interventions fall into one category or the other. Second and related, because the experimental nature of a treatment is its essence, the task of good policy is to ensure that the policy drawn neatly mirrors this nature. Being experimental is a fact of nature, which like other facts of nature can be known only through the proper method of factual investigation. Currently, the leading method for gaining such knowledge consists of the new "evaluation sciences," which are the sole legitimate scientific means to gain knowledge concerning effectiveness.[35] Thus, there is a slide down a slope in which a normative claim is transformed into a scientific question of fact: a normative question concerning distribution of resources becomes hinged on a scientific "evaluation" of effectiveness. Even the very name—"evaluation sciences"—evidences this confusion of fact for value. Third, the entire justificatory framework then metamorphoses to utilitarianism.[36] Because "scientific evaluation" becomes the prop necessary even to the normative arguments concerning distribution of resources, it then becomes justifiable to deny an individual's access to an intervention that has yet received the backing of that evaluation in order to create social incentives for the evaluation to occur. At this point the factual tail is wagging the normative dog: the need to obtain science becomes the highest value, to which all others must be subsumed, including any individual's particularistic claim to a biomedical intervention.

This transmogrification is evident in the way the experimental/nonexperimental distinction is administered. Consider, for example, its use in private insurance contracts. These contracts typically contain two interacting clauses. One defines the goods and services to be covered, usually stating that the insurance plan covers reasonable and necessary care. The second consists of a list of excluded services, and experimental treatments comprise one of those types. The two clauses work in conjunction with each other, because an excluded experimental treatment is not reasonable and necessary.

Questions of interpretation arise under these clauses because different arguments can be made whether a particular treatment is properly categorized as experimental or nonexperimental. Disputes concerning the coverage of high-dose chemotherapy with autologous bone marrow transplantation ("HDCT-ABMT") are aptly illustrative because the structure of the disputes is typical and has been made visible by much litigation and study. On the one hand, HDCT-ABMT diffused widely before well-conducted randomized trials existed. Relying on this evidence, patients and their caregivers have often successfully argued that the treatment is not experimental.[37] On the other hand, given the lack of phase III trials, insurance companies sometimes win these disputes. When they do, the definition of "experimental" that prevails becomes "that which has yet to be validated by phase III trials."[38]

Most often, resolution of these conflicts will depend on particular contractual language. Insurance contracts are usually drafted by insurance companies, and courts have long viewed them as vehicles designed to limit the insurer's liability by use of language that catches policyholders unaware. Courts are also aware that policyholders do not exercise market choice to the same extent as that exercised in unmediated transactions.[39] Most health insurance is employer provided. Employees usually receive a brochure that summarizes benefits and exclusions; they rarely read or even have access to the long insurance contracts themselves; they are often presented with a take-it-or-leave-it option by their employers; and contracts must be continually administered, with continuous changes in exclusions, because of changing medical technology and evidence concerning effectiveness. Finally, the insurer may focus just on its bottom line in a very competitive market, thereby ignoring the particular claims of particular policyholders. Accordingly, a standard rule of construction is that ambiguous language is construed in favor of the insured. Yet, courts are also increasingly aware that insurance funds are limited, and that there must be some social mechanism to make distributive choices. Because, for better or worse, we use market transactions as our social mechanism to make these distributive choices, this area is governed by the law of contract, and this balance is played out within and constrained by particular contractual language.

Relatively early (or extant poorly drafted) contracts contained (or contain) the typical exclusions for experimental treatment, but these clauses were construed against the insurer because the language did not (1) clearly commit the decision regarding medical necessity to the insurer;[40] (2) explicitly state the criteria by which to define experimental treatments;[41] or (3) clearly delineate the procedures that would be used in deciding how to categorize interventions as experimental or nonexperimental.[42] Over time, however, insurers are becoming more sophisticated in eliminating these ambiguities. Most important for our purposes, the ambiguity regarding the definition of medical necessity and experimental treatment is being eliminated in one of two ways. First, contracts contain longer and longer laundry lists of services deemed to be experimental; for example, HDCT-ABMT for breast cancer; HDCT-ABMT for Hodgkin's disease; and HDCT-ABMT for testicular cancer. These contracts eliminate the interpretive question altogether by specifying as exactly as possible particular interventions to be excluded.[43] However, given the inflexibility of such a device, and given its impracticality in the face of constant innovation and shifting scientific evidence, this strategy is not particularly viable.[44] Hence the second vehicle to eliminate ambiguity in interpretation is to commit the definition of experimental to a third-party decisionmaker that in turn relies on the evaluation sciences.[45] A particularly well-crafted example of such a clause, surely bound to be mimicked, is the following:

A . . . medical treatment is experimental or investigational: . . .

(2) if Reliable Evidence shows that the . . . medical treatment or procedure is the subject of on-going phase I, II, or III clinical trials or under study to determine its maximum tolerated dose, its toxicity, its safety, its efficacy, or its efficacy as compared with the standard means of treatment or diagnosis. . . .

Reliable evidence shall mean only published reports and articles in the authoritative medical and scientific literature; the written protocol or protocols used by the treating facility . . . or the written informed consent used by the treating facility. . . .[46]

One sees a similar movement in public insurance. Medicare can be used for illustrative purposes. Similar to private insurance contracts, the Medicare legislation does not contain an exhaustive list of covered services but instead provides for coverage of reasonable and necessary services.[47] A relatively lengthy list of services is expressly excluded,[48] but most exclusions occur because the Health Care Financing Administration (HCFA) or its contracting agents characterize a treatment as experimental.[49] Hence, a health care technology is reasonable and necessary if it has been proven to be "safe," "effective," not "experimental," "cost-effective," and "appropriate."[50]

The administrative procedures for making these terminations are fairly complicated but for our purposes three points are salient. First, usually HCFA and its contractors defer to technology assessments conducted by the Office of Health Technology Assessment (OHTA) within the Agency for Health Care Policy and Research or to technology assessments conducted in the private sector.[51] This practice is analogous to the incorporation of technology assessments within private insurance contracts and law, as previously described. Second, in OHTA's words, the "quality of the medical and scientific evidence is of paramount importance in formulating assessment conclusions. . . . Prospective, randomized controlled trials provide the most reliable medical and scientific evidence."[52] Other forms of evidence are ignored or heavily discounted. Again, the analogy to private insurance contracting is clear: the tendency is to define experimental treatments as those not yet validated by phase III trials.[53] Third, distributive considerations count for nothing in these determinations. What matters is scientific evidence concerning medical effectiveness and the need to save scarce budgetary resources to maximize the medical bang for all beneficiaries, a utilitarian mode of social choice that relies on scientific fact.[54]

To summarize, administration of the experimental/nonexperimental distinction is either becoming extremely formalized through the use of categorical exclusions or is being converted into a scientific question, decided by a third-party decision maker, which has no conflict of interest and uses the "objective" evidence provided by the evaluation sciences. Distributive questions, therefore, are completely decontextualized, converted into scientific questions, and decided on utilitarian grounds. Difficult normative issues such as the effect of a particular intervention on equality of opportunity, the just distribution of the costs of providing such an opportunity, the potential "social hijacking" of personal preferences, the particular situation and responsibility of a particular patient, and the like simply do not appear in the policy process. Rather, decisions are made on the basis of the fact of medical effectiveness alone or in combination with the fact of cost-effectiveness. This reduction of a normative question to a factual one occurs because statements in insurance contracts (or the *Federal Register*) incorporate statements generated in scientific papers, which in turn are incorporated by legal statements. Law, a form of public policy, therefore loses its normative edge as a vehicle for debating distributive justice. Put the opposite way around, scientific statements that capture the reality of effectiveness (or lack thereof) are made powerful because they are incorporated into a network of contractual statements, policy formulations written by the relevant public agencies, and statements made by courts of law. Moreover, there exists substantial evidence that this process of formulating policy discriminates against those persons least able to protect themselves: those without knowledge of their potential remedies and the resources to make use of those remedies.[55] Hence, a distinction that perhaps could be justified in a policy statement as a means of doing right—fostering equal opportunity—is being used to do wrong.

To be sure the factual question whether an intervention is an "enhancement" would differ from that used to decide if an intervention is "experimental." However, the process of reduction is likely to be similar. Just as the policy question regarding coverage for an "experimental" treatment—a normative issue that should be discussed in terms of equality or equity—has been reduced to a question of medical effectiveness, the policy question regarding coverage for an "enhancement"—likewise a normative issue that should be discussed in terms of equality or equity—will probably be reduced to a "biological" question concerning the intervention's impact on the "organism" and its physiologic "function." Thus an intervention that restores "normal physiological function" (a la Boorse)[56] would be a covered treatment; and an intervention that goes beyond such restoration would be deemed a noncovered "enhancement." While we in the Hastings Center Project might urge that the very definition of an enhancement should much more broadly canvass such considerations as the definition of a person, issues of justice, and contextualized questions concerning the impact on particular persons and various social activities, the policy process will likely reduce the relevant factors to facts of biology. The range of values deemed relevant will be narrowed, and the importance of considering a thick context will be ignored.

## The Enhancement / Treatment Distinction as a Tool of Medicine's Casuistry

We can perhaps summarize the argument of the previous section somewhat differently. The section was designed to indicate that a Hastings Center Project's policy statement, aimed at achieving developed principles of distributive justice, is likely to be torn from its ethical moorings and swept into a sea of cost containment and breathtaking insensitivity for questions of distribution and context. The conclusion can also be stated as follows: a policy statement written to affect the realm of value might instead end up displacing value. I do not intend thereby to indicate that we are foreclosed from attempting to affect the domain of value but instead that we might focus our efforts on different institutions because, if we try to influence the system of "policy," we will be swept into the issues of contract and public health insurance administration. In attempting to do right, we might as well tilt at windmills. Let's instead contrast the system of policy I just described with practices that might not so formalize, scientize, and "utilitarianize" our evaluative statements that they become unrecognizable to us.

I would hope that professional practices would constitute such an activity both because the clinical encounter is more likely to consider a wider range of values and because it is more likely to do so in a contextualized fashion than the policy process I just described. Hence I would argue that the treatment/enhancement distinction might be administered much differently in the patient-doctor encounter than in the insurance contract. While space here does not permit a full-blown account of the encounter, for present purposes we might analyze professional practices at two different levels, one "macro" and one "micro."

At the macro level we may, with Talcott Parsons, understand professionals as actively involved in the creation of value.[57] Parsons wrote that the "professional complex" is the "crucial structural development in twentieth-century society."[58] He maintained that the professions together comprise a system embodying ultimate values and are responsible for "society's cultural tradition . . . [,] for its perpetuation and . . . further development."[59] These conclusions followed as a logical matter from Parsons's answer to Hobbes's problem of social order.[60] Parsons employed a sociological reformulation of Kant's great question concerning knowledge: "given that society *does* exist, how is this possible?" Order is not considered to be problematic but is assumed. The economy, Parsons wrote, was the institutional embodiment of instrumental rationality.[61] However, if actors were oriented by instrumental rationality alone, their ends would be "random" and society an impossibility. Hence, because society does exists, there must be an institutional embodiment of "ultimate ends" which orders the otherwise disorderly ends of instrumental activity.[62] Parsons knew that somewhere in social structure there must be institutions that orient reason toward a universalized normative pattern.[63] Those institutions, he believed, include the professions.

We can adopt Parsons's insight concerning professional activities without following him into action theory, with its unsustainable account of motivation, and its metaphysical supposition that there exists some "cosmic glue" (my words) to hold society together.[64] Rather, we can locate the necessary normative binding in professional practices. Here we may discuss two aspects of medical practice to draw our contrast with the administration of a treatment/enhancement distinction in private and public insurance: the attention to the particular and a casuistry that has cognitive, affective, and normative dimensions.

Medicine may be described as an "art of the particular." This description is accurate in terms of both the "science" and the objects of beneficence or agency.[65] As Kathryn Hunter recounts so vividly in her ethnography of medical education, the process of education acculturates clinicians to assume the existence of, and therefore to seek, the irregular, rather than to presume and to find the regular.[66] Put differently, the process of clinical education inculcates in clinicians an implicit ontological commitment that the particular exists and is a good unto itself.[67] Accordingly, as Eric Cassell describes, clinical practice contextualizes patients: "clinicians treat particular patients in particular circumstances at a particular moment in time, and thus they require information that particularizes the individual and the moment."[68] Individuals are treated both as individual objects of biomedical science and as ends unto themselves.

In the ideal and often in action, these practices of the particular extend beyond the patient's biomedical situation to include that person's expression and values (as well as the practitioner's). As I've described elsewhere, "good doctoring *must* consist of attending to [an] entire story of illness, and it must be a process of inserting values and treating the whole person";[69] and, as Cassell in particular has excelled in showing, in treating patients as persons, good doctors attend to their patients' life histories, their characters and personalities, relationships, cultural backgrounds, roles, activities, fears, hopes, and values.[70] Moreover, *pace* Parsons's description of ultimate values residing in some nonempirical netherworld, this attention to the expressive and normative dimensions of care is part of medical practice—part of talking with patients.[71] As Sandy Tanenbaum has recently developed, talking with patients is the giving of an "account" to them, and this accounting necessarily includes all cognitive, expressive, and normative elements.[72]

To be sure, medical practice sometimes threatens to "biomedicalize" patients, thereby falling into the trap of scientism I described in the last section.[73] In a society and culture in which science is perhaps the most important badge of legitimacy, both organized medicine and individual practitioners have played the science card as a means to fend off challenges from other professionals seeking to capture "jurisdiction" of tasks in the division of labor,[74] to minimize the social dimensions of illness,[75] and to fend off challenges to their authority from lay individuals and institutions.[76] These assertions that "our knowledge is scientific" are used to justify not only the old experiential clinical science but also the new evaluative sciences discussed here.[77] Yet, we must always be sure to distinguish professionals' strategic descriptions of their work from the conduct of work itself; and we must be careful not to reify professional "knowledge" as "formal knowledge"[78]—a rational reconstruction of work as an "abstract, unsituated field of statements"[79]—but understand instead that knowledge is the practice of work itself.[80] Hence, when we pay attention to the work itself, we see, as Tanenbaum has written in her story of a communicative account,[81] and as ethnographic evidence shows,[82] that professional practice cannot and does not reduce to science.

In sum, administration of a treatment/enhancement distinction in professional practice stands a much greater chance of being highly contextualized and incorporating all of cognitive, aesthetic, and ethical practical knowledge,[83] than would administration of the distinction in the "policy" world of contracts and public health insurance. Perhaps then a Hastings Center Project statement regarding professional obligation would not be subverted beyond recognition—would not be reduced to a fragment—but would instead be taken up by professional practice as a coherent whole. Professionals do interact with lay values. Following the new sociological institutionalists,[84] we may describe norms as part of the resource environment from which professional practices draw and contribute in their "boundary spanning" activities.[85] Alternatively, and perhaps more fruitfully, we may describe professional practice as a cognitive, aesthetic, and normative casuistry in which a particular case is explored in all its cognitive, aesthetic, and normative richness and compared and contrasted with other cases personally known and with more generalized statements concerning the cognitive, aesthetic, and normative aspects of cases collectively known.[86] Either way, through a Hastings Center Project statement concerning professional obligation we might affect the discourse that Juengst has described,[87] and we might express such normative concerns as those raised by the other participants in this project.

## Conclusion

Policy discourse will determine when the use of a technology is a treatment or an enhancement. In our current social situation the most important discourse for the distribution of resources will be that of administering private insurance contracts and public insurance systems. This discourse will likely validate the reality of a treatment/enhancement distinction but either formalize it or hand over its delineation to the process of finding scientific fact. In this process the connection drawn between the distinction and an underlying normative theory will likely be severed, and the result will probably cause social wrong not social right. By contrast, administration of the distinction in the clinical encounter promises to be contextual and evaluative. Hence, we should direct social criticism of enhancements, not to policymakers, but to professionals in an attempt to influence the discourse concerning professional obligation.

## Acknowledgment

I am grateful for comments, suggestions, and encouragement from all participants in the Hastings Center Project "On the Prospect of Technologies Aimed at the Enhancement of Human Capacities," particularly Maggie Little and Erik Parens.

## NOTES

1. Eric T. Juengst, "What Does *Enhancement* Mean?" in this volume.

2. Dan W. Brock, "Enhancements of Human Function: Some Distinctions for Policymakers," in this volume.

3. Juengst, "What Does *Enhancement* Mean?"

4. Brock, "Enhancements of Human Function."

5. John W. Meyer and Brian Rowan, "Institutionalized Organizations: Formal Structure as Myth and Ceremony," *American Journal of Sociology* 83, no. 2 (1977): 341–63, at 342–43, 356–57.

6. Jeffrey L. Pressman and Aaron B. Wildavsky, *Implementation* (Berkeley: University of California Press, 1973).

7. Philip Selznick, *Leadership in Administration* (Evanston, Ill.: Row, Peterson, 1957).

8. Deborah A. Stone, *Policy Paradox: The Art of Political Decision Making*, 2nd ed. (New York: W. W. Norton, 1996), especially chap. 6.

9. Charles Taylor, "Interpretation and the Sciences of Man," in *Philosophy and the Human Sciences* (New York: Cambridge University Press, 1985), pp. 15–57; Charles Taylor, "Self-Interpreting Animals," in *Human Agency and Language* (New York: Cambridge University Press, 1985), pp. 45–76.

10. W. V. Quine, "Ontological Relativity," in *Ontological Relativity and Other Essays* (New York: Columbia University Press, 1969), pp. 26–68.

11. John W. Meyer, John Boli, and George M. Thomas, "Ontology and Rationalization in the Western Cultural Account," in *Institutional Structure: Constituting State, Society, and the Individual*, ed. George M. Thomas et al. (Newbury Park, Calif.: Sage, 1987), pp. 12–37.

12. Talcott Parsons, *The Structure of Social Action, Vol. I: Marshall, Pareto, Durkheim* (New York: Free Press, 1968), pp. 43–51.

13. Meyer and Rowan, "Institutionalized Organizations."

14. Paul J. DiMaggio and Walter W. Powell, "The Iron Cage Revisited: Institutional Isomorphism and Collective Rationality in Organizational Fields," *American Sociological Review* 48, April (1983): 147–60.

15. Richard W. Scott, "Unpacking Institutional Arguments," in *The New Institutionalism in Organizational Analysis*, ed. Walter W. Powell and Paul J. DiMaggio (Chicago: University of Chicago Press, 1991), pp. 164–82.

**16.** Richard Harvey Brown, "Social Reality as Narrative Text," in *Society as Text: Essays on Rhetoric, Reason, and Reality* (Chicago: University of Chicago Press, 1987), pp. 118–42. One could say "environment" instead of "field," but this sets up and fails to problematize an inside/outside distinction.

**17.** Roger Friedland and Robert R. Alford, "Bringing Society Back In: Symbols, Practices, and Institutional Contradictions," in *The New Institutionalism in Organizational Analysis*, ed. Walter W. Powell and Paul J. DiMaggio (Chicago: University of Chicago Press, 1991), pp. 232–63; Scott, "Unpacking Institutional Arguments."

**18.** Michel Foucault, "The Fantasia of the Library" in *Language, Counter-Memory, Practice*, ed. Donald F. Bouchard, trans. Donald F. Bouchard and Sherry Simon (Ithaca, N.Y.: Cornell University Press, 1977), pp. 87–109; and "Language to Infinity," in *Language, Counter-Memory, Practice*, pp. 53–67, at 66–67.

**19.** Michel Foucault, *The Archaeology of Knowledge* (New York: Pantheon, 1972).

**20.** Ann Swidler, "Culture in Action: Symbols and Strategies," *American Sociological Review* 51, April (1986): 273–86.

**21.** Bruno Latour, *Science in Action: How to Follow Scientists and Engineers Through Society* (Cambridge, Mass.: Harvard University Press, 1987).

**22.** Latour, *Science in Action*, p. 23.

**23.** Michel Foucault, *The Archaeology*: "Every statement is specified in this way: there is no statement in general, no free, neutral, independent statement; but a statement always belongs to a series or a whole, always plays a role among other statements, deriving support from them and distinguishing itself from them: it is always part of a network of statements, in which it has a role, however minimal it may be, to play" (p. 99).

**24.** Stone, *Policy Paradox*.

**25.** Theodore R. Marmor and William Plowden, "Rhetoric and Reality in the Intellectual Jet Stream: The Export to Britain from America of Questionable Ideas," *Journal of Health Politics, Policy and Law* 16, no. 4 (1991): 807–12.

**26.** Michael D. Cohen, James G. March, and Johan P. Olsen, "A Garbage Can Model of Organizational Choice," *Administrative Science Quarterly* 17, no. 1 (1972): 1–25.

**27.** By no means do I imply that material resources do not matter. The power of a policy is undoubtedly a combination of its connection to a linguistic scheme of justification and the affinities between that scheme and important things in life like material resources. One should always remember, however, that the material "situation" is never "given" directly to consciousness but is instead coextensive with the language we use to describe "it." Hence my definition of a policy statement—a description of what is and what ought to be—is intended to encompass a description of "material power." It might be fruitful to develop a descriptive scheme along the lines of Scott's three-layer cake analytic framework in which the symbolic or institutional realm recursively reacts with and is mediated by a technical realm, which in turn recursively reacts with and is mediated by the realm of adaptive and strategic—that is, purposive—behavior. Richard W. Scott, "The Organization of Medical Care Services: Toward an Integrated Theoretical Model," *Medical Care Review* 50, no. 3 (1993): 271–302. Yet we must remain sensitive to the fact that the technical realm cannot be analyzed as some existence separate from our language that describes it. In any event, I don't think that a Hastings Center Project's policy statement concerning enhancements will impose itself by virtue of power over material resources.

**28.** Analysis must describe "how the recurrent elements of statements can reappear, dissociate, recompose, gain in extension or determination, be taken up into new logical structures, acquire, on the other hand, new semantic contents, and constitute partial organizations among themselves." Foucault, *The Archaeology*, p. 60.

**29.** Jeffrey A. Alexander and Thomas A. D'Aunno, "Transformation of Institutional Environments: Perspectives on the Corporatization of U.S. Health Care," in *Innovations in Health Care Delivery: Insights for Organization Theory*, ed. Stephen S. Mick (San Francisco: Jossey-Bass, 1990), pp. 53–85; Scott, "The Organization of Medical Care Services."

**30.** Samuel Scheffler, *The Rejection of Consequentialism*, rev'd ed. (New York: Oxford University Press, 1994).

**31.** David M. Frankford, "Managing Medical Clinicians' Work Through the Use of Financial Incentives," *Wake Forest Law Review* 29, no. 1 (1994): 71–105; David M. Frankford, "Measuring Health Care: Political Fate and Technocratic Reform," *Journal of Health Politics, Policy and Law* 19, no. 3 (1994): 647–62; David M. Frankford, "Scientism and Economism in the Regulation of Health Care," *Journal of Health Politics, Policy and Law* 19, no. 4 (1994): 773–99; David M. Frankford, "Food Allergy and the Health Care Financing Administration: A Story of Rage," *Widener Law Symposium Journal* 1, no. 1 (1996): 159–265.

**32.** My discussion of the experimental/nonexperimental treatment distinction stems from my previous, much fuller and more elaborate work, Frankford, "Food Allergy." Nonetheless, my discussion also owes a substantial debt to Rand Rosenblatt's analysis in Rand E. Rosenblatt, Sylvia A. Law, and Sara Rosenbaum, *Law and the American Health Care System* (Westbury, N.Y.: Foundation Press, 1997), pp. 242ff.

**33.** David M. Eddy, "Benefit Language: Criteria That Will Improve Quality While Reducing Costs," *JAMA* 275, no. 8 (1996): 650–57; Mark A. Hall and Gerard F. Anderson, "Health Insurers' Assessment of Medical Necessity," *University of Pennsylvania Law Review* 140, no. 5 (1992): 1637–1712; John E.

Wennberg, "Innovation and the Policies of Limits in a Changing Health Care Economy," in *Technology and Health Care in an Era of Limits*, ed. Annetine C. Gelijns (Washington, D.C.: National Academy Press, 1992), pp. 9–33.

**34.** Eddy, "Benefit Language"; Peter. J. Neumann and Milton C. Weinstein, "The Diffusion of New Technology: Costs and Benefits to Health Care," in *The Changing Economics of Medical Technology*, ed. Annetine C. Gelijns and Ethan A. Halm (Washington, D.C.: National Academy Press, 1991), pp. 21–34.

**35.** John E. Wennberg, "What Is Outcomes Research?" in *Modern Methods of Clinical Investigation*, ed. Annetine C. Gelijns (Washington, D.C.: National Academy Press, 1990), pp. 33–46; Wennberg, "Innovations and the Policies of Limits."

**36.** Eddy, "Benefit Language"; Hall and Anderson, "Health Insurers' Assessment."

**37.** U.S. District Court, *Pirozzi v. Blue Cross-Blue Shield of Virginia,* Federal Supplement 741 (1990): 586–95; U.S. District Court, Adams v. Blue Cross/ Blue Shield of Maryland, Inc., Federal Supplement 757 (1991): 661–77.

**38.** U.S. Court of Appeals, *Harris v. Mutual of Omaha Co.,* Federal Reporter, 2nd ed., 992 (1993): 706–14; U.S. Court of Appeals, *Fuja v. Benefit Trust Life Insurance Co.,* Federal Reporter, 3rd ed., 18 (1994): 1405–12.

**39.** Rosenblatt, Law, and Rosenbaum, *Law*, pp. 242ff.

**40.** Illinois Court of Appeals, *Van Vactor v. Blue Cross Association,* North Eastern Reporter, 2nd ed., 365 (1977): 638–47.

**41.** U.S. Court of Appeals, *Pirozzi.*

**42.** U.S. Court of Appeals, *Reilly v. Blue Cross & Blue Shield United of Wisconsin,* Federal Reporter, 2nd ed., 846 (1988): 416–27.

**43.** U.S. District Court, *Wilson v. Group Hospital & Medical Services, Inc.,* Federal Supplement 791 (1992): 309–14; U.S. District Court, *Hilliard v. BellSouth Medical Assistance Plan,* Federal Supplement 918 (1995): 1016–28; U.S. District Court, *Bushman v. State Mutual Life Assurance Co. of America,* Federal Supplement 915 (1996): 945–54.

**44.** Jan Blustein and Theodore R. Marmor, "Cutting Waste by Making Rules: Promises, Pitfalls, and Realistic Prospects," *University of Pennsylvania Law Review* 140, no. 5 (1992): 1543–72; Hall and Anderson, "Health Insurers' Assessment."

**45.** U.S. Court of Appeals, *Harris;* U.S. Court of Appeal, *Fuja.*

**46.** U.S. Court of Appeals, *Harris,* p. 708.

**47.** U.S. Code, vol. 42, sec. 1395y(a)(1)(A).

**48.** U.S. Code, vol. 42, sec. 1395(a)(2)-(16).

**49.** Frankford, "Food Allergy."

**50.** Health Care Financing Administration, Department of Health and Human Services, "Medicare Program; Criteria and Procedures for Making

Medical Services Coverage Decisions That Relate to Health Care Technology," *Federal Register* 54, no. 18 (1989): 4302–18.

**51.** Frankford, "Food Allergy."

**52.** Agency for Health Care Policy and Research, Department of Health and Human Services, "Process for Health Care Technology Assessments and Recommendations for Coverage," *Federal Register* 58, no. 231 (1993): 63, 988–91.

**53.** Frankford, "Food Allergy."

**54.** In my previous work I described an instance in which a policy network was created by linking together the policy statements of a relevant medical community, OHTA, HCFA, the National Institute of Allergy and Infectious Diseases, and private insurers (see Frankford, "Food Allergy"). That lengthy case study cannot be replicated here. Suffice it to say that the description of the policy process was similar to that in this paper.

**55.** William P. Peters and Mark C. Rogers, "Variation in Approval by Insurance Companies of Coverage for Autologous Bone Marrow Transplantation for Breast Cancer," *NEJM* 330, no. 7 (1994): 473–77. Peters and Rogers found that variations in approval for HDCT-ABMT for treatment of breast cancer could not be explained by pretreatment clinical characteristics of the patients, the design or phase of the clinical trial, the year in which the request for coverage was made, or the patients' responses to previous conventional chemotherapy. They noted that in a substantial number of cases, patients gained a reversal of an insurer's initial denial of coverage after they hired an attorney, obtained media publicity adverse to the insurer, or obtained alternative resources for payment.

**56.** Christopher Boorse, "On the Distinction Between Disease and Illness," *Philosophy and Public Affairs* 5, no. 1 (1975): 49–68; and "Health as a Theoretical Concept, *Philosophy of Science* 44, no. 4 (1977): 542–73.

**57.** This discussion of Parsons is drawn from a much lengthier explication in a prior article. See David M. Frankford, "The Critical Potential of the Common Law Tradition," *Columbia Law Review* 94, no. 3(1994): 1076–1123.

**58.** Talcott Parsons, "Professions," in *International Encyclopedia of the Social Sciences*, vol. 12 (New York: Macmillan Press, 1975), pp. 536–47, at 545.

**59.** Talcott Parsons, "Some Problems Confronting Sociology as a Profession," *American Sociological Review* 24, no. 4 (1959): 547–59, at 547.

**60.** Talcott Parsons, "On Building Social System Theory: A Personal History," in *Social Systems and the Evolution of Action Theory* (New York: Free Press, 1977), pp. 22–76, at 69 n. 69.

**61.** Talcott Parsons, "The Professions and Social Structure," in *Essays in Sociological Theory*, pp. 34–49.

**62.** Talcott Parsons, "The Professions and Social Structure"; and "The Place of Ultimate Values in Sociological Theory," in *Talcott Parsons: The Early*

*Essays,* ed. Charles Camic (Chicago: University of Chicago Press, 1992), pp. 231–57.

63. Talcott Parsons, "The Motivation of Economic Activities," in *Essays in Sociological Theory*, pp. 50–68. More fully, Parsons built his action theory around the "act" as the basic unit of analysis. An act is the orientation of an individual's reason toward the accomplishment of an end. To formulate an end, an actor must interpret a "situation," which includes anticipated reactions of others. Because society exists—since actors do coordinate their activities—individuals must share an intersubjective understanding of the situation, including reciprocated understandings of what behavior is expected. Because it must therefore be true that actors' ends are coordinated, and because the orientation of reason toward "empirical ends"—instrumental rationality—cannot overcome the Hobbesian problem of order, reason must be both oriented instrumentally toward attainment of empirical ends and normatively toward attainment of "nonempirical ends," or, in other words, "ultimate values." Parsons, *The Structure of Social Action*; see David Sciulli, "The Practical Groundwork of Critical Theory: Bringing Parsons to Habermas (and Vice Versa)," in *Neofunctionalism*, ed. Jeffrey C. Alexander and Jonathan Turner (Beverly Hills, Calif.: Sage Publications, 1985), pp. 21–50. Embodied in culture, institutionalized in the social system, and internalized into personality, these ultimate ends suffuse empirical ends with a common motivational component such that actors share an intersubjective understanding of what types of interaction are appropriate in diverse situations—and the goals to be attained, the means available, and the standards to be applied in evaluating the fit between those means and ends.

64. Swidler, "Culture in Action."

65. For a longer description of this point, see Frankford, "Managing Medical Clinicians' Work."

66. Kathryn Montgomery Hunter, *Doctors' Stories: The Narrative Structure of Medical Knowledge* (Princeton, N.J.: Princeton University Press, 1991).

67. "How . . . particulars differ from one another in their diversity thus becomes as important as the characteristics they commonly share. Experience of a single entity over time is necessary for an understanding of that entity as a particular in all its distinctiveness, for its individual characteristics will not typically be inferable simply from what is known about the general—that is, commonly shared—characteristics of the type of entity of which it is an instance." Samuel Gorovitz and Alasdair MacIntyre, "Toward a Theory of Medical Fallibility," *Journal of Medicine and Philosophy* 1, no. 1(1976): 51–71, at 59–60. Further, particulars "have to be understood as wholes which maintain themselves in the world or fail to maintain themselves in the world. . . . Thus, not only does it make sense to speak of the good of such particulars; we cannot even study them without some reference to that good—without

indeed an ability to understand the particular from the perspective of its own *conatus*, its own striving toward its own good" (p. 61).

**68.** Eric Cassell, *The Nature of Suffering and the Goals of Medicine* (New York: Oxford University Press, 1991), p. 179.

**69.** Frankford, "Scientism and Economism," p. 789.

**70.** Cassell, *The Nature of Suffering*, pp. 37–46, 158–74.

**71.** Eric Cassell, *Talking with Patients, Vol I: The Theory of Doctor-Patient Communication* and *Vol. II: Clinical Technique* (Chicago: University of Chicago Press, 1985).

**72.** Sandra J. Tanenbaum, "Health Accounts and Communicative Power," *Journal of Health Politics, Policy and Law* 22, no. 1 (1997): 223–30; Sandra J. Tanenbaum, "Say the Right Thing: Communication and Physician Accountability in the Era of Medical Outcomes," in *Getting Doctors to Listen: Ethics and Outcomes Data in Context*, ed. Philip Boyle (Washington, D.C.: Georgetown University Press, 1998), pp. 204–23.

**73.** Elliot G. Mishler, *The Discourse of Medicine: Dialectics of Medical Interviews* (Norwood, N.J.: Ablex Publishing, 1984).

**74.** Andrew Abbott, *The System of Professions: An Essay on the Division of Expert Labor* (Chicago: University of Chicago Press, 1988).

**75.** Howard Waitzkins, "A Critical Theory of Medical Discourse: Ideology, Social Control, and the Processing of Social Context in Medical Encounters," *Journal of Health and Social Behavior* 30, June (1989): 220–39.

**76.** Eliot Freidson, *Professional Dominance* (Chicago: Aldine Publishing, 1970).

**77.** Gary S. Belkin, "The New Science of Medicine," *Journal of Health Politics, Policy and Law* 19, no. 4 (1994): 801–8.

**78.** Eliot Freidson, *Professional Powers: A Study of the Institutionalization of Formal Knowledge* (Chicago: University of Chicago Press, 1986).

**79.** Joseph Rouse, *Knowledge and Power: Toward a Political Philosophy of Science* (Ithaca, NY: Cornell University Press, 1987), p. 72.

**80.** Frankford, "Managing Medical Clinicians' Work."

**81.** Tanenbaum, "Health Accounts"; and "Say the Right Thing."

**82.** Byron J. Good, *Medicine, Rationality, and Experience: An Anthropological Perspective* (New York: Cambridge University Press, 1994), chap. 3; Byron J. Good and Mary-Jo Delvecchio Good, "The Meaning of Symptoms: A Cultural Hermeneutic Model for Clinical Practice," in *The Relevance of Social Science for Medicine*, ed. Leon Eisenberg and Arthur Kleinman (Boston: D. Reidel, 1980), pp. 165–96; Robert A. Hahn, "A World of Internal Medicine: Portrait of an Internist," in *Physicians of Western Medicine: Anthropological Approaches to Theory and Practice*, ed. Robert A. Hahn and Atwood D. Gaines (Boston: D. Reidel, 1985), pp. 51–111; Hunter, *Doctors' Stories*.

**83.** On ethics as practical knowledge, see James D. Wallace, *Ethical Norms, Particular Cases* (Ithaca, NY: Cornell University Press, 1996).

84. Meyer and Rowan, "Institutionalized Organizations."

85. David M. Frankford, and Thomas R. Konrad, "Responsive Medical Professionalism: Integrating Education, Practice, and Community in a Market-driven Era," *Academic Medicine* vol. 73, no. 2 (1998): 138–45.

86. I am developing the description of a cognitive, aesthetic, and normative casuistry in another work. David M. Frankford, "The Cognitive, Aesthetic, and Normative Casuistry of Medical Practice," in progress (199—). On casuistry generally, see Albert R. Jonsen and Stephen Toulmin, *The Abuse of Casuistry: A History of Moral Reasoning* (Berkeley, CA: University of California Press, 1988); Richard B. Miller, *Casuistry and Modern Ethics: A Poetics of Practical Reasoning* (Chicago: University of Chicago Press, 1996); and Wallace, *Ethical Norms.*

87. Juengst, "What Does *Enhancement* Mean?"

ANITA SILVERS

# A Fatal Attraction to Normalizing: Treating Disabilities as Deviations from "Species-Typical" Functioning

## Health Care as a Social Good

In the late twentieth century, (bio)medical ethics bifurcated into micro- and macrostudies, the former devoted to probing singular cases suffused with difficulties, the latter committed to finding some common good(s) to invoke so as to resolve hard as well as clear cases. Being clear about what kind of good health care represents, it was argued, enables us to decide who, in what circumstances, deserves it. To this way of thinking, while health is a personal good, health care is a social good. And it is not how to secure the former, but when to provide the latter, that is the challenge in morally difficult cases. Accordingly, macro-(bio)medical ethics developed an account of how to judge right and wrong in caring for patients, namely, by proposing what kind of health care, in what circumstances, a just society allocates.

Macro-(bio)medical ethics enthusiasts think that if we had a just system of health care, the right interventions would be evident. Once health care is cast as a social good, principles drawn from political morality will guide us in assessing the propriety and priority of various kinds of medical interventions. Just principles will enable us to see what should be provided for particular patients.[1] It is the nature of justice to illuminate the difference between obligatory and merely beneficial interventions, that is, between necessary treatment and salutary enhancement.

The latter may be privileging or not, depending on how the patient is circumstanced relative to other people. But the former is always equalizing, suggests Norman Daniels in presenting his immensely influential theory, which is meant to place the provision of health care on the firm foundation of democratic values that, by tradition, inform our public policy. What makes a medical intervention a treatment for Daniels, and what makes treatments equalizing vehicles is that they aim at preventing or remedying the disadvantages that people would otherwise suffer as the result of accident or disease.

> None of us deserves the advantages conferred by accidents of birth . . . It is . . . important to use resources to counter the natural disadvantages introduced by disease . . . This does not mean we are committed to the futile goal of eliminating or "leveling" all natural differences between people . . . [But] health care has normal functioning as its goal: it concentrates on a specific class of obvious disadvantages and tries to eliminate them.[2]

The notion of "leveling" that Daniels introduces here is a traditional theme in American political morality. Dissenting religious groups like the Quakers urged that society be arranged to show more respect for the commonalities of human nature, our essential humanity, than for artificial distinctions of class, caste, or role. Those committed to "leveling" were motivated by the conviction that all souls were equally valuable to God; therefore, all souls should have an equal voice in the community. The accidents of wealth and birth ought not to disadvantage people by limiting their opportunities for social participation.

Traditional leveling theories did not propose that all souls were identical, of course, but only that they have equal opportunity for community involvement and influence. Nor did these theories propose to eliminate the natural differences among people, only those accidental disadvantageous differences attendant on wealth and birth. Indeed, the argument for diminishing the importance assigned to wealth and birth (that is, to inherited rank) was that these socially constructed characteristics should not be allowed to obscure or impede the expression of natural talents and traits, the properties that naturally differentiate one individual from another.

In this tradition, Daniels's policy proposes that health care should eliminate, to the degree possible, the disadvantageous adventitious differences that occur when poor health impairs physical, sensory, or cognitive functioning. People should not be leveled in every way, for they naturally differ in skills and talents; only artificially disadvantageous differences should be eliminated. One of Daniels's important contributions to the traditional discussion is to suppose us to have become so proficient in the practice of medicine that the disadvantageous differences attributable to unrepaired poor health are artificial—as when people remain in ill health due to an unjust system of distributing effective medical interventions. If the disadvantages associated with poor health are thus as much a social as a natural product, our "leveling" tradition urges that deficiencies in people's functioning that result from poor health should be remedied so as not to diminish the opportunities their skills and talent would otherwise secure for them. Daniels writes:

> We are obliged to help others achieve normal functioning, but we do not "owe" each other whatever it takes to make us more beautiful, strong, or completely happy.[3] . . . The uses of health care that most of us believe we are obliged to make available to others are uses that maintain or restore normal functioning, not simply any use that enhances our welfare. . . . This distinction between the treatment of disease and disability and the enhancement of otherwise normal appearance or capabilities is reflected in the health care benefit packages of nearly every national health insurance system, whether public or mixed, around the world.[4]

And as he concludes in another text, "If people have a higher-order interest in preserving . . . opportunity, . . . then they will have a pressing interest in maintaining normal species functioning by establishing institutions—such as health care systems—that do just that."[5]

On this (bio)ethical emendation to political morality, medical treatment has a public value because it is an instrument of the state's commitment to protect all citizens equally against arbitrary disadvantage. Interventions that merely enhance the welfare or well-being of individuals in respects in which they are not disadvantaged do not have a similar public value.

> The central function of health care services is to keep us functioning as close to normal as possible. Since maintaining normal functioning protects the range of opportunities open to people, by providing an appropriate set of health care services, we make a significant contribution to preserving equality of opportunity.[6]

Treatments, then, are those interventions that are used to reduce or remedy whatever disadvantage is occasioned by abnormal functioning that is associated with ill health. Because treatments are so defined, they are necessarily equalizing, in the sense that to be treatments they must be aimed at preventing or rectifying disadvantageous functioning and, consequently, at reducing or eliminating a specific kind of disadvantage the patient has in comparison with normally functioning individuals. Treatments can be prospective as well as retrospective on this view. For example, as the purpose of vaccination programs is to prevent some individuals from becoming disadvantaged by the sequelae of disease, to vaccinate children against polio or measles is to treat them.

Treatments are processes, however, and a process that has a definitive objective may not always succeed in reaching it. For example, it can be accurate to describe what we do in relation to our students as "educating them" even if some of the students are not educated. Similarly, treating someone may not always succeed in restoring that individual to the desired mode and/or level of functioning. But the key to a medical process's being a treatment is the plausibility of our casting it as a procedure to eliminate a disadvantage by restoring functioning.

For example, breast reductions often count as treatments now that a convincing case for the disadvantageousness of very large breasts is made; for example, she can't buy clothes that fit, she can't run because of their weight, they make her an object of derision in the workplace. But we can imagine social contexts in which it is much harder to make this case. If women custom-made their own clothes, rarely ran (because society insisted it isn't lady-like to run) and never, never pursued careers in the workplace (because fathers and husbands did not want women to work outside the home), it would be harder to argue that the breast reduction procedure remedies disadvantages rather than merely increases a woman's comfort. For in that context women would not normally engage in the performances the procedure rehabilitates or restores. But this does not totally resolve the issue, for some women may desire to transform the roles females are permitted to adopt and so may argue that breast reductions remove one of the barriers to women's assuming such roles. They might argue that in their case breast reduction is not merely a means of enhancing the welfare of large-breasted women with unfashionable preferences for comfort over sexual attractiveness; rather, it responds to a legitimate need to eliminate a social disadvantage.

Considerations such as these raised by the breast reduction procedure lead to questions about the neutrality of appealing to normal fashions of functioning. Sometimes, people who function in the normal fashion are, for that very reason, confined to roles that are disadvantageous and detract from their flourishing. This restriction has surely been the case for women in societies in which women have been assigned to disadvantageous roles on the ground that their normal fashion of functioning prohibited their achieving in more highly valued roles. Since the goal of treatment is to remove disadvantage, but normal fashions of functioning can be disadvantageous, why does Daniels believe that (maintaining or restoring) functioning in a normal fashion is the standard for determining whether an intervention is a treatment?

## Normalizing

Whether or not I am an individual whose disadvantage is reduced because I receive treatment, social arrangements providing for the reduction of undeserved disadvantage occasioned by physical, sensory, or cognitive dysfunction are for the public good, Daniels says, and thus for my good insofar as I am a community member. Daniels comments:

> I abstract from the special effects that derive from an individual's conception of the good. This level of abstraction seems appropriate given our search for a measure of the social importance, for claims of justice, of impairments of health. My conclusion is that we should use impairment of the normal . . . as a measure of the relative importance of health care needs.[7]

Because treatment is a public good, the condition which occasions or invites it should be objective and independent of transitory social accidents, Daniels believes.[8] What he takes to be the natural difference between normal functioning and functioning corrupted by illness or accident suggests to him a fixed and objective, and therefore an appropriately public, standard for ascertaining the occasions when treatment should occur. "Where we can take as fixed, primarily by nature, a generally uncontroversial baseline of species-typical functioning," we can show, he thinks, "which principles of justice are relevant to distributing health care services."[9] Daniels thinks that the way the species typically functions constitutes a natural and therefore a neutral standard to which the public can assent.

First, all "people have a fundamental interest in protecting their share of the normal range of opportunities."[10] Second, maintaining "normal species functioning" is necessary to protect this high-order interest persons have in maintaining a normal range of opportunities: "Life plans we are otherwise suited for and have a reasonable expectation of finding satisfying or happiness-producing are rendered unreasonable by impairments of normal functioning. . ."[11] Third, and crucial to Daniels's argument, is his assumption that normal functioning is natural and thereby neutral in that the criteria for determining what functioning is normal are biological rather than social. "The basic idea is that health is the absence of disease, and diseases (I here include deformities and disabilities that result from trauma) are deviations from the natural functional organization of a typical member of a species."[12] This step of the argument is critical, for it is here that we are told why not functioning as people typically do is disadvantageous. When disease is the reason individuals do not function in typical fashion, their resulting performances must be inferior to those that issue from individuals whose natural functional organization has not been corrupted by disease.

Of course, this argument leaves open what counts as being diseased. Daniels thinks that the line between disease and its absence generally is noncontroversial and publicly ascertainable through the methods of the biomedical sciences.[13] Others argue to the contrary, of course. For example, Susan Sherwin points out that some elements of women's lives—for instance, menstruation, pregnancy, menopause, body size and feminine behavior—have been medicalized and treated as diseases because they have been viewed as disruptive of normal functioning.[14] In the same vein, genetic conditions that result in what we think is inferior functioning are equated with disease. These examples suggest that not disease but functioning in the normal fashion is the controlling notion here.

John Rawls, on whose theory Daniels relies to scope out justice in health care and other domains, gives us a political perspective on normal functioning. He remarks:

> [A] person is someone who can be a citizen, that is, a fully cooperating member of society over a complete life . . . [F]or our purposes . . . I leave aside permanent physical disabilities or mental disorders so severe as to prevent persons from being normal and fully cooperating members of society in the usual sense.[15]

Here is an additional reason to think of a policy of normalizing functioning as an instrument that secures the ends of democratic political morality. For on the view that being a well-functioning individual is critical to performing the social responsibilities of citizens, normalizing is seen as qualifying functionally defective individuals for citizenship by repairing them so they can execute the usual social interactions and sustain common social responsibilities. To do so they must conduct themselves normally and be able to comply with other people's natural expectations of them. For whoever cannot perform competently as a cooperating and contributing and, therefore, an equal, social partner is fully neither citizen nor person.

## The Right to (Normalizing) Treatment

The prescription is clear: although interventions that enhance a patient's functioning so that it departs from what is normal may be advisable for the patient when they enhance the patient's welfare, only interventions that normalize command a broader social warrant. That is because normalizing interventions restore or maintain individuals as cooperative, contributing citizens.

To understand what is at stake, we should notice that at least two aspects of functioning, the mode and the level, affect whether the performance of a function is normal. A function's mode is the way it is accomplished. To illustrate, the normal mode in which we execute the function of reading a document is by seeing the text. This function can be executed in other ways, for instance, tactilely if the text is brailled, aurally if the text is scanned into a computer with a voice output screen reader. These alternative or adaptive modes may support a normal level of functioning. If the individual is adept, she may still read at normal speed and comprehension. Or she may function in the alternative mode above or below the normal level. According to Daniels, restoring individuals who have suffered impairment of functioning through illness or accident to the normal mode and level of functioning takes priority. If treatment fails, the next step is adaptation.

> One important function of health care services . . . is to restore handicapping dysfunctions (e.g., of vision, mobility, and so on). The medical goal is to cure the diseased organ or limb when possible. When a cure is impossible, we try to make function as normal as possible, through corrective lenses or prosthesis and rehabilitative therapy. But when restoration of function is beyond the ability of medicine per se, we begin another area of services, nonmedical support services.[16]

It is important to notice that this system gives mode of functioning precedence over level of functioning. On it, we first attempt to restore the patient's ability to function in the customary mode, seeing or walking or hearing the way other people do. Afterward, if a cure proves impossible, we apply prostheses—corrective lenses, artificial limbs and physical therapy, hearing aids, and lipreading lessons. These prostheses may restore the patient to the typical level of functioning (or enhance it, remember the Bionic Man) but not (quite) to the normal mode: lipreading requires that those engaged in dialogue face each other, artificial limbs demand both stump and prosthesis maintenance, corrective lenses must be put on and removed.

Parenthetically, Daniels complains that social support services are allocated fewer resources than restorative treatment. Given Daniels's account up to this point, his preferred explanation is curious. He hypothesizes:

> Yet for various reasons, probably having to do with the profitability and glamor of personal medical services and careers . . . as compared with services for the handicapped, our society has taken only slow and halting steps to meet the health care needs of those with permanent disabilities.[17]

It is odd for him to think that the reason society does not provide sufficient social support services is because doing so is not sufficiently personally profitable or glamorous for professionals. His own account provides a more persuasive explanation, namely, that the initial response to defective functioning, which consequently has first call upon resources, is restorative treatment. On his own account, normalizing interventions do and should take precedence over interventions with any other kind of impact because their outcomes are assigned a higher social or political value.

This priority is because normal functioning appears to be a firm and impersonal, yet compelling, goal, whereas we have no reliable standard of what counts as satisfactory if an individual does not function normally. Normal functioning is a clear standard as well, Daniels supposes, because to determine what normal function is, we need only observe the natural functional organization of human beings. This task, he says "falls to the biomedical sciences . . . since claims about the design of the species and its fitness to meeting biological goals underlie at least some of the relevant functional ascriptions."[18] So neither the predominant functional modes nor the modal functional levels are artifactual, he thinks. Because the functioning that typifies a species seems so expressive of its nature, species-typical functioning appears to be a self-justifying standard, nature's way of deducing how we ought best to conduct ourselves given what kind of creature we are.

Further, what could be a more modest and natural expectation of individuals than the prospect of functioning as their species typically does? Given these considerations, all individuals equally are found to have a natural stake in social arrangements designed to prevent or repair anomalous conditions that interfere with species-typical functioning. Concomitantly, relatively few individuals would have an interest in preserving or promoting any specific functional anomaly or singularity.

So it seems as if the broadest-based public support very naturally will go to social arrangements that reduce whatever anomalies or singularities hinder adherence to the species-typical functional standard.

The protean character of two of the notions pivotal to Daniels's argument, namely, those marked by the designations "natural" and "normal," is striking. Absent the suggestion that these are virtually interchangeable characters, in that our normal fashions of functioning are those that are natural rather than acquired, there would be no obvious connection between normalizing modes of functioning and equalizing opportunity. For there is nothing unusual in equally healthy people experiencing vast differences in the opportunities available to them, nor in people in different states of health enjoying similar scopes of opportunity. But our species has evolved a natural functional organization so well-suited to realizing these goals, Daniels thinks, that an individual's falling away from this organizational standard by not functioning normally cannot help but diminish his or her options for desirable achievement.

What apparently is important here is not actualized opportunities. Rather, what is supposed to be equalized is the amplitude of options that each individual has available for achieving our species' biological goals. It might seem, then, that nature determines what normal species functioning is (a biological premise) and in doing so specifies the mode and level of functioning individuals need to exhibit if they are to enjoy meaningful equality of opportunity (a social conclusion).

Yet when we probe more deeply into Daniels's account of just health care, we find that it is a social rather than a biological value that informs and validates reparative interventions. Indeed, it is not even a sociobiological value, for rather than surrendering individual benefit to the species' collective evolutionary good, the value to which Daniels appeals is simply an extension of the liberal sociopolitical commitment to preserving equal access to opportunity for the individual.

Daniels's standard is biological, but the principle that implements it clearly is not. For biology tends to eliminate truly dysfunctional individuals, not repair them. The principle that advises us to restore people's normal functioning through health care is also not an expression of an impersonal sociobiological drive of individuals to maintain their species. At most it is an intersubjective principle with the potential to unify the personal interests individuals have in maintaining a competitive position. It suggests that we should be suspicious of claims that there is a biological mandate that accredits policies of normalizing people by restoring them to typical or familiar modes and levels of functioning.

"Normalizing" has a passionate component, of course, namely, our tribal preferences to congregate with individuals like ourselves. But our attraction to the company of our counterparts, which can be intense, is not usually thought to justify a public commitment to allocate resources to repair those who do not measure up. Simply avoiding or excluding those who fall away from the common standard is the usual concomitant of our passion for congregating with those who most resemble us. The difficulty with thinking of a policy of normalizing as a component of democratic political morality becomes even more evident when we notice that normalizing is sometimes privileging rather than equalizing. For instance, interventions that help some individuals more closely approach species-typical functioning may deprive, disadvantage, or otherwise reduce opportunities for individuals who function normally already. And, as we saw when we considered the value of breast reductions, making normalizing our policy can also be unfair if it worsens the position, or otherwise oppresses, the very individuals whose functioning it purports to repair by, for instance, depriving them of anomalous but effectively adaptive alternative modes of functioning.

We should be wary of policies that cloak privileging certain fashions of functioning in the mantle of the "normal." Normalizing then is not the self-evidently right thing to do. Nor can we justly allocate health care without careful attention to the circumstances of whoever is normalized.

## What Is Being Normal?

How useful is the concept of normalizing in warranting medical interventions considered case by case? Whether, in fact, there is much clarity about what normalizing is raises a second kind of concern about its compatibility with egalitarian ends, for there is a tendency to equivocate to a dangerous degree as to the meaning of this admittedly circumstantial standard. In "The Meaning of Normal," Phillip Davis and John Bradley comment:

> Medicine uses the word normal to express . . . various meanings. . . . In medicine, normal can refer to a "defined standard," such as normal blood pressure; a "naturally occurring state," such as normal immunity; . . . "free from disease," as in a normal pap smear . . . "balanced" as in a normal diet, "acceptable" as in normal behavior, or it can be used to

describe a stable physical state. In all these meanings . . . normal is used to describe an "ordinary finding" or an "expected state." But medicine allows another meaning . . . that differs significantly from the ordinary. [M]edicine has come to understand normal as a "description of the ideal." . . . Defining the norm as an ideal leads to significant problems. . . . Disease and ill health are a normal part of the human condition. The constant pursuit of health . . . leads easily to blaming those who bear the burden of illness. . . . More important . . . are the problems that result from defining variation from the ideal as "abnormal." . . . Accepting the ideal as the norm begs the question of how uncommon something must be to be considered abnormal.[19]

Current practice assigns pathological conditions the role of being signifiers of unhealth. But because it is not cost-effective to intervene wherever pathology occurs—that is, to conduct an all-out campaign to normalize all parts of all people—current practice takes a further conceptual step by identifying some departures from the norm as incapacitating, while others are tolerated as benign. Davis and Bradley observe: "When the ideal is taken as the norm, variation becomes defined as disease—an especially peculiar circumstance insofar as much variation has no particular clinical significance or biological consequence."[20]

Christopher Boorse suggests that it is usual on current practice to assess departures from the norm as warranting intervention if they cause death, disability, discomfort, or deformity.[21] Interventions are made not on the ground of the rarity of the condition but rather its disruption of function. But while death indubitably is incapacitating, disability, discomfort, and deformity need not always be so. To define such conditions as necessarily dysfunctional and consequently as demanding intervention begs the question.

Surely, any measure used to sanction intervention should distinguish what is not normal and thereby harmful from what is not normal but merely unusual or anomalous. This is to avoid justifying every culture's every intercession into anomalies regarded by that culture as pathological. For instance, for the Punan Bah of Borneo, the birth of twins is a greater social disgrace than the birth of a spastic, blind, or retarded child. It is so socially disturbing and disadvantageous a condition that it is also dysfunctional, for after twin births, one twin always dies (unless it is given to another family living distantly enough to achieve the concealment of its twinhood).

## Normal Quality of Life

To distinguish such prescientific practices to remove anomalies from modern medical practices to abate defects in individuals, Dan Brock very usefully attempts to say more about the damage that departures from being normal can do. In *Life and Death* (1993) Brock correctly eschews offering an absolute standard for knowing when medical intervention properly remedies abnormality.

> The dominant conception of the appropriate aims of medicine focuses on medicine as an intervention aimed at preventing, ameliorating, or curing and thereby restoring, or preventing the loss of, normal function or of life. Whether the norm be that of the particular individual, or that typical in the particular society or species, the aim of raising people's function to above the norm is not commonly accepted as an aim of medicine of equal importance to restoring function up to the norm. Problematic though the distinction may be, quality of life measures in medicine and health care consequently tend to focus on individuals' or patients' dysfunction and its relation to some such norm.[22]

How does dysfunction present itself as a diminution of quality of life? Brock observes: "At a deep level, medicine views bodily parts and organs, individual human bodies, and people from a functional perspective."[23] But what one must go on to grapple with is the difficulty of connecting, let alone commensurating, different kinds or levels of functional descriptions. An increasingly familiar component of medical judgment, so-called quality of life scales are meant to quantify well-being to determine for what and on whom health care dollars are best expended.

Brock cites such a "Quality of Well-Being Scale"[24] to illustrate a discussion about containing high-cost but low-benefit treatments. Of almost equal weight on the scale are what are designated as the patient's physical activity level, namely, how competently the patient executes the performances of daily living, and (assigned just slightly more importance) the patient's functional level, that is, what the patient achieves through engagement in daily life performances.

But these rankings do not reflect the subtleties of what can be achieved despite impairment. In the physical activity category of the scale Brock cites, mobilizing by walking, albeit with a feeble gait, ranks higher than using a wheelchair to be mobile. But which mode actually facilitates mobility more effectively is not nearly as clear as this scale makes it out to be. For while wheelchair users are more limited in the types of sites they can access, they exceed the customary level in respect to the speed at which and distance from where they travel to those sites. Individuals who mobilize by walking can climb into many more types of sites but only those they have the time and stamina to reach.

The physical activity category assesses the modes individuals adopt to perform a function and then assigns the patient a rank that reflects the degree to which his mode of functioning diverges from the customary mode. Walking very feebly more closely resembles our customary mode of mobilizing than wheeling very vigorously, so the individual who uses the former mode is assessed as enjoying a higher quality of life than the individual who uses the latter. On the other hand, the functional category addresses interactions between the patient and the environment. For whether someone who uses a wheelchair can get into a car or use public transportation, for instance, is as much a question about the availability of appropriately designed vehicles as it is about the patient.

This abstracting from complex differences between kinds of limits suggests that the scale is more responsive to the mere fact of an individual's being limited than to how functionally devastating or benign the limit might be. We should discount any scale that arbitrarily fixes the relative effectiveness of different modes of performing any function, any scale that equates what is most common with what is best, and equally any scale that illegitimately naturalizes such rankings by appeal to biological imperatives. For mechanically aided functioning is not necessarily inferior to unassisted activity, no more is driving twenty miles to be disparaged as the crutch of subnormal hikers, and no more than manually signed communication is categorically inferior to speech. In general, we should mistrust any scale of well-being that purports to measure life's quality by comparing modes of functioning in a way that obscures how modes that are not the common fashion can nevertheless be fully functional.

Moreover, we should distrust any summative process that commensurates fixed and variable elements while disregarding the contexts to which the latter are relativized. The degree to which either personal or environmental limitations result in social limitations—that is, prevent an individual from normal social achievement like having a family and earning a living—is the outcome of complex interactions between the individual's limits and the limits of his or her environment. It is therefore difficult not only to predict the degree to which, but also to comprehend the process whereby, physical or environmental dysfunction leads to social dysfunction.

Brock himself recognizes that even serious physical limitations do not always lower quality of life if the disabled persons have been able or helped sufficiently to compensate for their disabilities so that their level of primary functional capacity remains essentially unimpaired; in such cases it becomes problematic even to characterize those affected as disabled.[25]

As the individuals Brock describes just prior to writing this passage are persons without arms and legs, this remark is revealing. If their eating, driving, painting pictures, raising a family—the functions of a good life that Brock portrays them as achieving—makes it problematic to describe them as disabled, then underachieving must be part of the definition of disability. And if being disabled is tied so firmly to lowered achievement, then even very marked deviation from species-typical functioning has only circumstantial connection to disability.

For it is far from clear that deviations from normal functioning mean either lowered productivity or decreased quality of life. Far from being the natural way of conducting ourselves, the modes of functioning that typify our species may merely be ways of doing things that are preferred by the dominant classes and to which we have therefore become accustomed. To the extent that this preference is the case, policies of normalizing, however well-intentioned, threaten not to equalize but to preserve existing patterns of functional dominance and privilege, a problem exacerbated by an absence of clarity in the practice of medicine in regard to establishing what is normal.

## A Social Instrument for Normalizing

Accordingly, we need to clarify the nature and consequences of a public policy that gives expression to a mandate to normalize, an inquiry that I propose to pursue by exploring an analogous sphere, the domain of education. At least two reasons compel us to consider what we can learn from comparing analogous practices in education and health care. First, our current public policy intersects the two domains by legislating entitlements to preventative health education and rehabilitative special education within the public educational system. Indeed, a surprisingly large amount of what Daniels describes as basic health care needs are served by the public education system. Given that it is an egalitarian value, equalizing opportunity, that ultimately justifies the allocation of health care on Daniels's view, he is relatively expansive in delineating what is needed "to maintain, restore, or provide functional equivalents (when possible) to normal species functioning. These include adequate nutrition and shelter, safe and unpolluted living and working conditions, preventative and rehabilitative personal medical services, and nonmedical personal (and social) support services."[26]

Using public education to deploy preventative, curative, and rehabilitative health care services is, of course, a very familiar practice. During the past century, day and residential schools in this country have, to give some examples, enforced preventative vaccination policies; promoted safe, sanitary, unpolluted, and tobacco-free living; ensured that children are given the basic principles of nutrition; instructed students about maintaining the health of their reproductive systems; identified and referred children in need of reparative care for vision, hearing, and other impairments; and offered rehabilitative speech, psychological, and other therapies, or adaptive education for blind children or deaf children, on their premises. Second, Daniels himself not only finds the analogy between educational and medical benefit apt but relies on it to argue for social support for (universal) health care:

> [T]here is an important analogy between health care and education. Both are strategically important contributors to fair equality of opportunity. Both address needs that are not equally distributed among individuals. Various social factors . . . may produce special learning needs; so too may natural factors, such as the broad class of . . . disabilities. . . . [E]ducational needs, like health care needs, differ from other basic needs . . . Both at the national level and in many states, legislation to meet special educational needs . . . is justified by reference to the opportunities it protects.[27]

Daniels construes education as a reparative technology, while Brock[28] describes it as an enhancement technology. The difference between their views lies in whether, as Daniels thinks, our educational priority should be to teach all children the knowledge and skills normally required to be participating, contributing citizens, or whether, as Brock has it, our educational priority should be to advance the widest array of children's cognitive abilities so as to nourish their different talents and give each appropriate personal opportunities for flourishing. In education as in health care, then, there is a question about the priority to assign to engendering normal functioning.

## The Ascendancy of the Normal

In this regard, the battles that raged for nearly a hundred years about how best to educate deaf children provide an opportunity to assess the benefits of giving priority to normalizing. In the late nineteenth century, educators of the deaf bifurcated into two camps, one that passionately supported and one that vehemently opposed educating deaf children in the language of manual signs. Each charged the other with protracting the dysfunctionality of deaf people and consequently with unfairly constricting their opportunity. At the heart of this debate lay another divide, namely, an unbridgeable chasm that separated two very different beliefs about the relationship between biology and opportunity. As Douglas Baynton writes in *Forbidden Signs: American Culture and the Campaign Against Sign Language*: "The real battle (over sign language) was fought on a . . . rarefied plane, encompassing such questions as the larger purposes of education in a democratic and industrializing society . . . and the locus and character of cultural authority in America. Indeed, occupying a central place in the fight was a late-nineteenth century debate over the nature of nature itself."[29]

That deaf individuals talk by means of manual signs has been recognized since antiquity. Plato refers to this mode of communicating in the Cratyllus (422e). In the early part of the nineteenth century manual sign language schools were established to equalize deaf people's access to the Word, understood to be the conveyance of that moral and religious knowledge which is the goal of human imagination, intelligence, and understanding. Because manual signing was thought to rely on natural symbols that were self-interpreting, Sign was believed to engage the intelligence directly and lucidly, and to stimulate the moral sense. Sign therefore was the instrument to repair deaf people's dysfunction and permit them to develop to greatest perfection. America followed Europe in becoming fascinated by signing. Teachers were imported to systematize and disseminate the gestural communication used by the deaf in this country.

Manualists considered deaf people to be a singular class, distanced from the transient fashions of speech and therefore less corruptible, out of the ordinary, remarkable, unique. Citing such eighteenth-century sources as Daniel Defoe and Denis Diderot, Lennard Davis writes in *Enforcing Normalcy: Disability, Deafness and the Body* that, for different reasons and in different respects, both the blind and the deaf were often thought to exhibit certain heightened and purer sensibilities than the ordinary person.[30] Far from being roleless, deaf people were assigned a special place in the eighteenth- and early nineteenth-century imagination.

But, as Baynton observes, "by the late nineteenth century, natural-ness as an ideal was being challenged and eventually was not merely defeated but colonized by the competing ideal of 'normality.' "[31] For one thing, naturalness had lost its status as a trait independent of and superior to the artifice, convention, and craft characteristic of social organization. "This intellectual and indeed moral shift in American culture was crucial to the reversal in attitudes toward sign language and the deaf community," Baynton adds.[32]

An 1884 speech by oralist Alexander Graham Bell shows how naturalizing the preferred behaviors of the dominant class propelled a program of normalizing, where this meant conforming the behaviors of deaf children to those of the hearing majority: "I think we should aim to be as natural as we can. I think we should get accustomed to treat our deaf children as if they could hear. . . . We should try ourselves to forget that they are deaf. We should teach them to forget that they are deaf. We should . . . avoid anything that would mark them out as different from others."[33]

By 1899 we find the President of Amherst College, John Tyler, folding the mantle of science around these normalizing practices. Tyler assured a convention of oralists that America would "never have a scientific system of education until we have one based on . . . the grand foundation of biological history. . . . [T]he search for the . . . goal of education compels us to study man's origin and development."[34] (This is not unlike the appeal to science Daniels makes in saying that biological science shows us how the natural functional organization of the species is a design "that permits us to pursue biological goals as social animals.")[35] Such scientifically based or biologized education would maintain the functional strategies that seemed to place speech higher on the scale of evolutionary development than the expressive gestures of lower pri-mates. The political morality of the time made it a moral and social obligation to increase the opportunities of both deaf signers and gesticu-lating foreigners by repairing them, a duty which a scientific system of educating them in the language and communication behaviors of the dominant class could help discharge.

It is important to understand that the fundamental division here is between competing ideas of what organizes a well-ordered society. The eighteenth-century's ideal of individualized moral perfection had given way to an ideal of communal or social participation by people who functioned dialogically in common in the public sphere. Where once language's highest function had been to engage individuals with ideas understood as transcendent sources of right belief and right conduct, now its most important use was to engage people with one another in productive commercial and civic interaction.

Arguing against the idea that deaf people could flourish with a language of their own, an oralist insisted: "To go through life as one of a peculiar class is the sum of human misery. No other misfortune is comparable to this."[36] This thought typifies the shift of priorities from personal to social improvement, and the correlated elevation of the importance of collective over idiosyncratic individualistic identities.

This urge to create fair opportunity by leveling the players rather than the playing field is a theme which has come more and more to dominate American egalitarianism over the past hundred years. What is striking is that systematically "normalizing" how deaf people communicate (and many other rehabilitation strategies) may amplify anomalous individuals' opportunities by making them more fit to pursue these, but concomitantly may make them less able to perform alternatively or adaptively. By devaluing alternative or adaptive modes of functioning, the policy transgresses liberal political theory's requirement that the state remain neutral between different citizens' ideas of the good life. Oralism's defense of its violation of this dictum was that, until deaf individuals communicated and consequently contributed in the normal mode, they could not be qualified for the protection due citizens.

Normalizing is played out in both medical and educational programs that intervene to repair or restore or revise members of nondominant groups so they qualify as citizens. In education, normalizing has been expressed as a mandate to assimilate the children of immigrant families to the dominant culture, and to impose the practices and preferences of males upon females. In being presented with arguments for normalizing deaf children, the public was invited to decide whether the management of "deaf schools" should be awarded to hearing people who promised to assimilate deaf children. By allocating resources to educational techniques intended to normalize deaf people, public policy imposed a conception of the good under which they did not flourish. We need to ask now whether there are some people who may not flourish, or whose well-being will be compromised, if normalizing similarly warrants and consequently guides the allocation of resources that go to health care.

## A Cost/Benefit Assessment of Normalizing

Normalizing has costs. If maintaining or restoring normal function is of such public significance that a system of benefits is made available for this purpose, it is hard to resist supposing that those whose functioning is anomalous ought to acknowledge the system by assigning the same priority to being restored. Baynton reminds us: "Oralism meant that many deaf people had access only to limited or simplified language during the crucial early years of language development."[37] For fear they would fall back to communicating in a more convenient but "abnormal" or "unnatural" way, deaf children were often not taught to write unless they had mastered intelligible speaking. This practice left a legacy of reduced literacy among deaf people.

Interventions that reduce rather than expand already limited functionality surely extract too high a price, but such is the history of oralism in the education of the deaf. "Oralism failed," Baynton concludes, "and sign language survived, because deaf people themselves chose not to relinquish the autonomous cultural space that their community and language made possible." That is, for many people who do not hear, the opportunity of communicating fully within a limited group appears to be more satisfying, more equalizing and more meaningful than the opportunity of communicating in a limited way with the larger community. This is not to say that all deaf and hard of hearing people make this choice, but merely to point out that the alternative to normalizing often is not a limitation of full functioning but merely a limitation in the expanse of environment in which one functions successfully.

Tribalism, our partiality for interacting with those most like us, undoubtedly influences us to assign preeminence to (the appearance of) normalcy. But to the degree it corrupts the positive balance of benefits over personal and public costs, serious questions about whether the policy of normalizing compromises fair opportunity rather than promotes it must be addressed.

The Canadian Health Care system's intervention in the cases of children born with missing or shortened limbs because their pregnant mothers took thalidomide illustrates this last point. In their treatment, appearing more normal was the priority, so much so that large public sums were expended to design dysfunctional painful prostheses which actually decreased their dexterity and mobility. They could walk with these, but only painfully and slowly. Reminiscent of the oralist ban on signing, they were forbidden to roll or crawl, although these modes offered much more functionality, at least within their home environments.

The direction of resources to fund artificial limb design and manufacture rather than wheelchair design was influenced by the supposition that walking makes people more socially acceptable than wheeling does. As the children became independent adults, less vulnerable to the aggressive elements of institutionalized health care, they discarded the dysfunctional prosthetics in favor of wheelchairs, some made to their own designs. Here is another case (among many such examples I could adduce) in which the tyranny of the normal cost anomalous individuals to sacrifice an effective level of functioning at the alter of social preference for a particular mode of functioning, and in so doing compromised rather than equalized their opportunities.

We should not underestimate the coercive potential of policies that validate a particular mode of functioning by directing resources to efforts to restore that mode. When oralism dominated in schools for the deaf, deaf children could either try to lip read and speak, or have no education at all. For the Canadian children with no usable lower limbs, mechanical limbs were the only mobility option offered because policy directed the resources to institutions that designed and engineered limb-like prostheses, not wheelchairs. More generally, then, to commit public policy to restoring individuals to species-typical modes of functioning diminishes public recognition of, and consequently resources for, alternative modes of functioning.

So far, we have seen that normalizing equalizes opportunity primarily for those who can be maintained in or restored to the image of the dominant group. But no natural biological mandate nor evolutionary triumph assures that the functional routines of this group are optimally efficient or effective. Rather, the members of this group have the good fortune to find themselves in a social situation that suits them.

For others, there is the choice of limited functionality in an ordinary environment, or ordinary functionality in a limited environment. How much opportunity need be absent from the former alternative, or sacrificed by the latter, depends upon how expansive the nonhostile environment can be made. Replacing staircases with spiral ramps for wheelchair users, adding captions to televised programs for deaf viewers, alt-tags to computer icons so that the screen readers used by people who are blind can identify them, all these make the constructed environment less hostile to and more inclusive of people who function in anomalous, alternative, or adaptive modes.

The main ingredient of being (perceived as) normal lies in finding or creating social situations that suit one. Contrary to Daniels's claim, normalizing is no self-warranting process that deserves the allocation of resources because it furthers democratic values. For individuals with disabilities, for example, such values are better advanced by developing social environments accustomed to people like one's self. The record of their history does not support assuming that broad social or moral benefits accrue to normalizing interventions. The attractiveness of warranting health care interventions that maintain/restore normal functioning on the ground that they are instruments of justice therefore appears to be much dimmer than the initial enthusiasm of macro-(bio)medical ethics for normalizing suggests.

## Disability, Self-Respect, and Lowered Quality of Life

Nothing said so far should be interpreted to mean that interventions to maintain or restore familiar modes of functioning never enhance individuals' welfare. But as we have seen, no clear difference in social benefit, or strict difference in obligation, separates these interventions, ones Daniels would call treatments, from interventions that enhance already average functionality. Then why is functioning normally of such value that maintaining or restoring this level becomes a decisive standard?

A critical component of a good quality of life, Dan Brock says, depends on each of us measuring our capacities and capabilities favorably against the standard of normal human functioning.[38] That is, whether we function normally or not influences how we rate ourselves in comparison to others and consequently affects our confidence and self-esteem. This observation suggests that the paramount benefit of being normal is to maintain the psychosocial well-being of tribalism.

Brock may well be correctly describing a self-reflective process our current cultural standards promote. But this is not sufficient to defend the process as reliable or otherwise reasonable. We have seen that normal functioning is hardly a firm and reliable mark of the quality of our performance. Indeed, it is so fragile a standard that Brock worries about how easily a program of genetic intervention might shatter it. Brock, and others, are alarmed by the potential genetic intervention has for disrupting our confidence in the standard of normalcy.

First, if we manipulate genes to raise the level of performances that typify our species, any pretense that typical functioning is a natural rather than manipulated standard vanishes. Heretofore, a social structure that privileges some people to control communications and construction to suit themselves has determined what modes of functioning are considered normal. Henceforth, a social structure that privileges some people to influence genetic research and the allocation of genetic interventions might determine what levels of functioning become normal. What is feared is that our current confidence in a firm and impersonal, because natural, standard of normality will be undermined by a new and widespread recognition of seemingly normal functioning as being merely the artifactual expression of the interests of whichever members of our species are positioned to deploy technology.

Will such an eventuality constrict rather than enlarge opportunity? Applying genetic technology that increases disparities of access to opportunity initially appears to be inconsistent with a democratically informed health care system, regardless of how much personal welfare the applications might bestow. Consequently, justice appears to advise constraining, or even prohibiting, these important broad applications of genetic technology.

For instance, genetic intervention could result in improving how some people function, so that someone who performs at a level that was comfortable for his species-average parents might find that the naturally good genes he inherited from them are surpassed by great genes installed in his competitors as a compensatory or even as a privileging measure. Constraining applications of this technology so that no individual can acquire an abnormally large number of desirable characteristics may seem advisable. But it is hardly an implementable policy, for the desirability of many of our characteristics is itself provisional and dependent on environment. Whether, and how, adding specific characteristics benefits the recipient—whether it privileges, equalizes, or just makes one more comfortable—must be decided with regard to the context in which the patient will function.

Brock is also concerned about whether, as we come to understand genetic structures accurately enough to identify the potentially anomalous functioning consequent on every species' member's inheritance, some members of the species will find themselves devalued by their own futures. Although performing splendidly at the time, they will be labeled, and consequently marginalized, as being at greater risk than others of deteriorating function. So, for instance, those at risk of Alzheimer's would be rejected as mates by whoever wanted the services of a spousal caretaker, while employers desiring to keep medical insurance costs down would not hire individuals genetically disposed to developing various kinds of cancer.

With the widespread use of genetic testing, he worries:

> [P]eople who feel healthy and who as yet suffer no functional impairment will increasingly be labeled as unhealthy or diseased. . . . For many people, this labeling will undermine their sense of themselves as healthy, well-functioning individuals and will have serious adverse effects both on their conceptions of themselves and the quality of their lives.[39]

Notice that, at this point, the idea, rather than the reality, of nonnormal functioning has become the signifier of whether someone is equally well off, or is advantaged or disadvantaged in comparison to others. This observation suggests that it is one's psychosocial rather than physical functioning that is most vulnerable to variations from accustomed states or normal prognoses—that is, to deviations from what is typical of our species. Brock describes how this occurs: "Generally it is when we have noticed an adverse effect or change in our normal functional capacity that we contact health care professionals and begin the process which can result in our being labeled as sick or diseased. . . ."[40] Brock thinks an adverse outcome of a genetic test could trigger this same process, though deterioration in physical functionality has not been and perhaps never will be manifested. Here being labeled as likely to become nonnormal initiates psychosocial processes that themselves are dysfunctional. The perception of being disadvantaged thus precedes and causes, rather than follows upon, dysfunction.

So the standard constructed to identify who is disadvantaged itself becomes the facilitator of disadvantage. Applying genetic technology then is merely the occasion, not the cause, of an unjust constriction of opportunity. It need not be categorically constrained for fear it will do so. For notice now how the disconnect between actually functioning differently and being disadvantaged has opened even wider. In the case about which Brock worries, individuals are functioning normally but are disadvantaged by having a significant potential, perhaps never to be actualized, for anomalous functioning. Here the social convention of the sick role, rather than the realities of effective performance, determines what modes and levels of functioning are advantageous, indifferent to advantage, or disadvantageous.

The prospect of increasing the power of the standard of species-typical functioning to consign individuals to the sick role undoubtedly is alarming. However, it is not the standard, but the science that could extend its applications, that is typically attacked. So Adrienne Asch and Gail Geller express their concern that "the Human Genome Initiative could turn out to make 'species-typical functioning' a guide to joining or remaining part of the human community."[41]

To counter these worries about genetic research, we should turn from policies of normalizing to approaches that make us more receptive to alternative ways of functioning. The strategy of protecting against discrimination those who function differently, are genetically disposed to function differently in future, or are perceived as functioning differently is of great help here. The 1990 Americans with Disabilities Act offers one strategic example; another is the recent stream of legislation protecting patients against disclosure of the results of genetic testing.

### *"Black, Yet White: a Hated Color in Zimbabwe"*[42]

If we initiate proper protections against the tyranny of the normal, genetic technologies that greatly increase our repertoire for adaptation have a far greater potential for promoting justice than for compromising it. They have this potential because they open new avenues for social compensation. But our discussion so far advises our approaching this technique for improving disadvantaged individuals with some caution. To illustrate, I want to consider the wisdom of changing the pigmentation of individuals whose birth color is a disadvantage.

There is wide agreement that resolving the American color problem by turning African Americans white is unjust. But our democratic intuitions about turning white people black are much less assured. In the United States, albinism occurs in about one out of every twenty-thousand births; in some parts of Africa, in one out of every one thousand to two thousand. "In Africa, far more than on any other continent, [albinism] is a lifelong curse. . . . As white-skinned men in a black society, they are shunned and feared as the products of witchcraft," writes Donald MacNeil Jr. in a front page story[43] in the *New York Times*. Should white Africans resident in Africa be turned black if this is the normal pigmentation of the members of their tribe? If normalizing is the instrument of justice, we have a pressing reason to help them do so.

Let us suppose that emerging genetic technology will soon permit us to intervene. Let us also suppose that for biological, cultural, and economic reasons, including the widespread incidence of the genetic factors that contribute to the condition (one individual out of seven is a carrier of a recessive gene for one or another of the types of albinism), screening to eliminate the birth of people with albinism in Africa proves impractical. Let us suppose, too, that we develop a series of relatively uncomplicated gene therapies so that neonates with albinism are enabled to produce the requisite enzymes or other factors related to skin-color that their type of albinism makes them lack.

Does a just health establishment owe it to African infants with albinism to widely distribute this therapy, making it as available as, for instance, are a variety of treatments such as the polio vaccine, or cleft-lip and club-foot corrective surgery? It is imaginable that such a policy would find opposition, on grounds of fairness, in the very sites where albinism is most common, namely, in those parts of Africa referred to in the *New York Times* article. For in those places, according to the article, people with albinism are thought of as a model minority who are seen as being more intelligent and successful than their black brothers and sisters.

Although their intelligence tests fall in the same range as their sisters' and brothers', as a group, Africans with albinism develop higher capabilities, possibly as an adaptation to their physical limitations. It is hypothesized that their light-sensitive and deficient vision, and their sun-sensitive skin, restrict them to contemplative rather than active life styles, which encourage them to be more studious and which qualify them for more education and more respected and better remunerated careers. By having fewer opportunities, they are more easily focused on ones that would be more advantageous for anyone. Parenthetically, Africans with albinism may benefit to some extent economically from the respect traditionally accorded those thought to be powerful witches. In regard to the entire spectrum of opportunities for social participation, Africans with albinism participate less in tribal or communal opportunities but participate at a higher than normal rate in those that are educational and economic.

## Normalizing, What Priority?

Given these realities, ordinarily pigmented but poor Africans could easily think that it would be unfair to expend scarce resources to increase pigmentation in their brothers and sisters with albinism. This group does well enough as it is, and so treating the genetic anomaly that creates their disadvantage in regard to some forms of socializing might enhance the already highly competitive level of functioning of this successful minority. On the other hand, because they overcome some of their natural disadvantage, do Africans with albinism then not deserve additional social support, namely, a program of reparative gene therapy? Are they owed nothing to remedy their social isolation?

So is turning white skin black any more pressing a social responsibility than deploying surgical skills to bring prodigiously down-turning or up-turning noses into conformity with the fashionably modest nose, or filling acne scars with collagen? Because there may be no firm answer as to whether a health care intervention does or does not level social advantage, we often cannot deduce from principles of justice whether a medical intervention effects treatment or enhancement. Consequently, even in a just system—indeed, especially in a just system—this distinction is unlikely to guide us in determining what should be provided for particular patients.

Of course, health care's primary mission is to keep us functioning. That Africans with albinism are ostracized socially argues for compensatory intervention regardless of whether, all things considered, they are a group that already succeeds economically. But what kind of intervention is most just remains an issue. To justly liberate group members' many talents, its members could be altered to better satisfy the expectations that pervade their social environment. On the other hand, altering the environment to better support their flourishing may correct their disadvantage equally well.

Neither the personal and social costs, nor the logistical difficulties attendant on each alternative, can be ignored in the course of developing compensatory policies. In the event biological alteration is the preferable policy, neonates with albinism would have to be identified and their families convinced to accept intervention. Arguably, the increase in physiological benefit—reducing vulnerability to the ravages of the sun—added to the significant social benefit of eliminating a provocation for discrimination, might sway the balance. On the other hand, social arrangements for distributing protective clothing and suntan oil might also adequately improve personal welfare, but only if the social environment is organized to embrace those who appear deviant, if it is, in fact, an environment reformed so as not to turn anomaly into dysfunction.

This last consideration remains too much neglected by prominent strategists of health-care justice. As we have seen, our normal modes and levels of functioning are, to an extent that often goes unrecognized, socially relative constructions rather than independent biological facts.

Adjusting the environment so anomalous individuals can better flourish can be as compensatory as leveling them. Moreover, enhancing individuals or their groups by magnifying their exemplary performance in some domains can, under some circumstances, sometimes compensate for there being barriers to their performance in other domains of functioning. Wherever strategies that equalize the amount of opportunity individuals have available rather than homogenize the kinds of opportunities they can access are feasible, there is even less reason to suppose that restoring anomalous individuals to normal modes of functioning is a better instrument of justice than enhancing the effectiveness of their anomalous modes.

In positing justice as the regulatory ideal of health care, macro-(bio)medical ethics initially proposed a deductive model on which principles of justice would inform our picking out and prioritizing those medical interventions that further equality. Interventions that qualify as treatments because they aim effectively at restoring normal function were, on this model, to take precedence in the allocation of resources. As we have seen, however, endorsing maintenance or restoration of normal functioning as the standard for allocation can itself, all too readily, prolong disadvantage. Macro-(bio)medical ethics must therefore overcome its fatal attraction to normalizing in order to open itself to other strategies for advancing justice.

## Acknowledgment

An early version of this paper was presented to the "Work in Progress" seminar at Stanford University's Center for Biomedical Ethics. I would especially like to thank Dr. Patrick Fox of the University of California at San Francisco and Dr. Rachel Cohon of Stanford University for their very thoughtful and helpful comments.

## NOTES

**1.** Norman Daniels, "Justice and Health Care," in *Health Care Ethics: An Introduction*, ed. Donald VanDeVeer and Tom Regan (Philadelphia: Temple University Press, 1987), pp. 290–325 at 290–93.

**2.** Daniels, "Justice and Health Care," p. 312.

**3.** Norman Daniels, Donald Light, and Ronald Caplan, *Benchmarks of Fairness for Health Care Reform* (Oxford: Oxford University Press, 1996), pp. 25–26.

4. Daniels, *Benchmarks*, p. 21.

5. Daniels, "Justice and Health Care," p. 301.

6. Daniels, *Benchmarks*, p. 41.

7. Daniels, "Justice and Health Care," p. 306.

8. Daniels, "Justice and Health Care," p. 300.

9. Daniels, "Justice and Health Care," p. 303.

10. Daniels, "Justice and Health Care," pp. 306–7.

11. Daniels, "Justice and Health Care," p. 301.

12. Daniels, "Justice and Health Care," p. 302.

13. Daniels, "Justice and Health Care," p. 303.

14. Susan Sherwin, *No Longer Patient* (Philadelphia: Temple University Press, 1992), p. 179.

15. John Rawls, "Justice as Fairness: Political not Metaphysical," *Philosophy and Public Affairs* 14 (1985): 223–51 at 233–34.

16. Daniels, "Justice and Health Care," p. 318.

17. Daniels, "Justice and Health Care," p. 318.

18. Daniels, "Justice and Health Care," p. 302.

19. Phillip Davis and John Bradley, "The Meaning of Normal," *Perspectives in Biology and Medicine* 40(1), Autumn (1996): pp. 68–77 at 69–70.

20. Davis and Bradley, "Meaning," p. 70.

21. Christopher Boorse, "Concepts of Health," in *Health Care Ethics: An Introduction*, ed. Donald VanDeVeer and Tom Regan (Philadelphia: Temple University Press, 1987), pp. 359–93, at 368.

22. Dan Brock, *Life and Death* (New York: Cambridge University Press, 1993), p. 297.

23. Brock, *Life and Death*, p. 297.

24. Brock, *Life and Death*, p. 346.

25. Brock, *Life and Death*, p. 307.

26. Daniels, "Justice and Health Care," p. 304.

27. Norman Daniels, *Just Health Care* (Cambridge: Cambridge University Press, 1985), p. 46.

28. Dan Brock, "Enhancements of Human Function: Some Distinctions for Policymakers," this volume.

29. Douglas Baynton, *Forbidden Signs: American Culture and the Campaign against Sign Language* (Chicago: University of Chicago Press, 1996), p. 107.

30. Lennard Davis, *Enforcing Normalcy: Disability, Deafness and the Body* (Verso, 1995), p. 53, 57–59.

31. Baynton, *Forbidden Signs*, p. 110.

32. Baynton, *Forbidden Signs*, p. 110.

33. Baynton, *Forbidden Signs*, p. 136.

34. Baynton, *Forbidden Signs*, p. 36.

35. Daniels, "Justice and Health Care," p. 302.

36. Baynton, *Forbidden Signs*, p. 145.

37. Baynton, *Forbidden Signs*, p. 151.

38. Dan Brock, "The Human Genome Project and Human Identity," in *Genes and Human Self-Knowledge: Historical and Philosophical Reflections on Modern Genetics*, ed. Robert Weir, Susan Lawrence, and Evan Fales (Ames, Ia.: University of Iowa Press, 1994), p. 18–33, at 31.

39. Brock, "The Human Genome," p. 29.

40. Brock, "The Human Genome," p. 29.

41. Adrienne Asch and Gail Geller, "Feminism, Bioethics and Genetics" in *Feminism and Bioethics*, ed. Susan M. Wolf (Oxford: Oxford University Press, 1996), pp. 318–50, at 330.

42. Donald MacNeil, "Black, Yet White: A Hated Color in Zimbabwe," *New York Times*, 2/9 (1997): pp. 1 and 6.

43. MacNeil, "Black, Yet White," p. 1.

KATHY DAVIS

# The Rhetoric of Cosmetic Surgery: Luxury or Welfare?

Medical interventions in the human body are burgeoning. From open heart surgery to organ transplants to gene therapy and the new reproductive technologies, the possibilities for technological enhancement seem almost unlimited. While these interventions are supposed to prolong life, improve health, and/or enhance well-being, in practice, they are often dangerous, expensive, and morally problematic. In recent years, controversies have emerged about the desirability of such extensive medical meddling in the human body and life cycle.

One such controversy concerns cosmetic surgery, which is by far the fastest growing medical specialty, both in the United States and abroad. Millions of people—most of whom are women—flock to plastic surgeons each year to have their faces "lifted," their breasts "enhanced" or their tummies "tucked," as the operations are euphemistically called.[1]

Despite the enormous popularity of cosmetic surgery, the operations are invariably painful, have myriad, often permanent side effects,[2] and frequently leave the recipient in worse shape than before the operation. Feminists have been unanimously critical of cosmetic surgery as a practice that reproduces ideologies of sexual inferiority.[3] Women are instructed that their bodies are never good enough—too fat, too flat-chested, too old, or too "ethnic." Cosmetic surgery is regarded as a particularly pernicious expression of the disciplinary regimes of the feminine beauty system—a way, quite literally, too "cut women down to size."

Cosmetic surgery is not only controversial for feminists, however. The medical profession has increasingly found itself in the position of having to justify performing dangerous surgical interventions on otherwise healthy bodies. Moreover, in the wake of a rapidly aging population and the state's inability to meet even basic health care needs, medical insurance companies have to warrant funding expensive operations for what is often seen as a luxury problem.

In this paper, I want to explore some of the debates that have emerged in the Netherlands concerning cosmetic surgery. The Netherlands has the somewhat dubious distinction of being the only country in the world to actually include cosmetic surgery in its basic health care package. Any individual who could demonstrate that she or he needed cosmetic surgery could have it paid for by national health insurance. As a result, more cosmetic surgery was performed per capita in the Netherlands than in the United States.[4] This cosmetic surgery "boom" was, financially speaking, bad news for a welfare system that was already having difficulties meeting even the most basic health care needs of its rapidly aging population. Cuts had to be made and cosmetic surgery, along with other medical practices, became the subject of heated debate. Was it necessary for the welfare of a particular individual or was it a luxury item that does not belong in the basic health care package?

Based on the problems that emerged in trying to justify cosmetic surgery in the Netherlands as well as the outcome of the debate, I will discuss some of the limitations of a moral rhetoric based on equality, universality, and distributive justice for justifying cosmetic surgery—and, by implication, other controversial medical practices like *in vitro* fertilization (IVF), gene therapy, and so-called smart drugs. This having been done, I will argue that an ethic which draws on a rhetoric of difference, care, and solidarity can provide a better starting point for coming to terms with the ethical issues that these practices raise.

## The Rhetoric of Health Care

In different health care systems, different rhetorical strategies are drawn upon to justify, defend, or criticize controversial medical technologies and practices. As David Frankford has argued, health care policy is not based on the incontrovertible facts of the case.[5] It is a social process by which actors "grab" their arguments from those available to them within a justificatory framework and deploy them in such a way that they will resonate with what has already been constituted as feasible, reasonable, and desirable. The rhetoric which is used in such debates depends, among other things, upon the way health care is organized.

In a market system—like the United States—health care is provided (at least until quite recently) on a fee-for-service basis and medical services tend to be distributed on the basis of availability. Specialists are "free" to provide services, just as patients are "free" to choose the health care they desire, provided they can pay for it. In principle, patients are consumers with equal rights to health care. In practice, public access is not guaranteed and many services are, therefore, only available to the affluent.

In a market system, the rhetoric used to justify controversial medical practices and technologies revolves around the issues of risk, malpractice, and informed consent. The medical profession, and more indirectly, the regulatory bureaucracy is accountable for practicing medicine in such a way that risks are kept at a minimum. Patients are free to use dangerous or experimental medical procedures, provided they know what they are getting into. Once informed, patients are left to "choose" for themselves.

In a welfare system—like the Netherlands and most western European countries—health care is provided by the state and medical services are distributed on the basis of necessity. In principle, a patient has a right to any form of health care he or she needs. Health care is not simply a privilege to be enjoyed by those who can afford it, but an entitlement for every citizen, regardless of his or her social position. In practice, however, many services are too expensive for the state to fund. The most common problem in the European welfare model of medicine is that requests for medical services and technologies are increasing at about the same rate as government funds for such services and technologies are decreasing.

In a welfare system, the rhetoric used to justify medical practices and technologies revolves around issues of welfare vs. luxury and how to make choices in heath care. The medical profession shares at least some of the responsibility for the overall expense of the health care system. The main focus of medical accountability is whether a particular practice or technology is a luxury or really necessary for citizens' health and well-being. A discourse of need shifts attention from risk to whether a particular medical service or procedure is "really" necessary in a context of scarcity. There is generally an implicit or explicit consensus that "unnecessary" services cannot be included in the basic health care package and must, therefore, be abandoned or made available through other means.

An example is the recent "Choices in Care" debate in the Netherlands. This debate was a broad, government-sponsored campaign to convince Dutch citizens of the necessity of making decisions about the availability of medical procedures, technologies, and medications in the Netherlands. A governmental task force—the Dunning Commission—was also established to develop normative criteria for evaluating health care services.[6] They came up with the following: Is the service necessary? Is it effective? Does it do what it is intended to do? Can the service be provided through private means? It was assumed that by assessing the health care services presently covered by national health insurance, services could be removed from the basic health care package, thereby reducing health care expenditure.

## The Dutch Case

Prior to 1980, cosmetic surgery was a small, but acceptable branch of plastic surgery. Like any other medical practice, it was included in the basic health care package, provided the surgeon thought it was necessary. Initially, plastic surgeons did not justify performing cosmetic surgery in terms of the patient's physical characteristics. Instead, they reiterated that appearance is a source of psychosocial problems and can cause an unacceptable degree of damage to the person's happiness and well-being. They defended cosmetic surgery patients against charges of vanity or hypochondria. On the contrary, there were "psychological" reasons for wanting surgery, such as bereavement, feelings of inferiority, and sexual frigidity. Children with "jug ears" run the risk of being teased by their classmates and women with sagging breasts may be afraid to go swimming with their children. Problems with appearance can lead to antisocial or even suicidal behavior. Cosmetic surgery is not a luxury, they reasoned, but a necessity for alleviating a specific kind of problem. The term "welfare surgery" was born.[7]

Cosmetic surgery became problematic, however, in the early 1980s, when there was a dramatic increase in cosmetic surgery with nearly every type of operation doubling in frequency.[8] For a welfare state already in crisis, this expansion was bad news. In an attempt to stem the flow of applicants for cosmetic surgery, plastic surgeons, together with medical inspectors from the national health insurance companies, were asked to develop guidelines for making decisions about which operations were necessary and which were not. They began by establishing three categories of cosmetic surgery that would be eligible for coverage by national health insurance:

- a functional disturbance or affliction (for example, eyelids which droop to such an extent that vision is impaired),
- severe psychological suffering (for example, the patient is under psychiatric treatment specifically for problems with appearance), and

• a physical imperfection which falls outside a "normal degree of variation in appearance" (that is, the patient's appearance does not meet certain aesthetic standards as determined by the medical inspector).

The first two categories were unproblematic as the criteria could be derived within medical discourse. Moreover, patients rarely applied for cosmetic surgery on the basis of severe psychological suffering because it meant bringing a report from a psychiatrist. The majority of the cosmetic surgery recipients fell under the third category, however, and it was this category—"outside a normal variation in appearance"— that proved to be something of a headache for the national health insurance system and, indirectly, for the plastic surgeons.

Initially, medical experts, in collaboration with the national health insurance system, attempted to develop guidelines for abnormal appearance. They looked for criteria that could be objectively observed, classified, and applied to all candidates for cosmetic surgery. Undeterred by the adage that "beauty is in the eye of the beholder," they originally seemed convinced that appearance—as another feature of the body— could be assessed scientifically.

Some problems did, indeed, seem to be amenable to classification. For example, ears could be measured in centimeters; that is, how far they protruded from the side of the head. A breast lift was indicated if the "nipples were level with the recipient's elbows." A "difference of four clothing sizes between top and bottom" was sufficient indication that a breast augmentation or liposuction was in order. Although these criteria may not sound exactly scientific, they did have the advantage of being clear-cut. Other criteria were much more vague. For example, for a face-lift, the person's countenance should look "10 years older than her or his chronological age." A sagging abdomen which "makes her look pregnant" provided reason enough for performing an abdominoplasty ("tummy tuck"). Eyelid corrections were justified if "the person looks like he or she has been out drinking all evening."

Such were the criteria that were developed in order to decide "objectively" whether or not an operation was necessary and, therefore, deserved full medical coverage. The fact that the criteria seemed based more on common sense than science is only part of the problem. More seriously, they proved totally inadequate in the practical context of deciding which kinds of cosmetic surgery should be covered by national health insurance. I can illustrate this inadequacy with an example concerning a relatively minor form of cosmetic surgery: the removal of tattoos.

Initially, it was agreed that tattoo removal should not be covered by national health insurance. The argument was that tattoos are put on voluntarily at the recipient's own expense and should, therefore, be taken off the same way. This seemed fairly straightforward until a large number of Moroccan immigrant women began coming in to have their tattoos removed. The medical inspectors began to falter, wondering— as they put it—just how voluntary the tattoos of these women had actually been. Whereas tattooing in Holland was apparently considered part of the individual's right to experiment with her or his body, tattooing in Morocco was viewed as a practice performed under coercion—a symbol of cultural constraint. The reasoning was that if such tattoos had not been done voluntarily and were, furthermore, detrimental to migrant women's integration into Dutch society and, by implication, their well-being, then an exception had to be made. Thus, the criterion was changed: surgical removal of tattoos was covered by national health care, provided the recipient was not Dutch-born.

No sooner had this new guideline been established, when the next problem arose in the form of a highly publicized rape case in which the rapist had drugged his victim and tattooed his name on her stomach. When she came in to have the name of her assailant removed surgically, she was denied coverage on the grounds that she was Dutch-born. The victim filed a complaint and the press got hold of the incident, much to the embarrassment of the medical inspectors. After several behind-closed-door meetings, national health decided that, once again, an exception should be made.

The tattoo episode is but one example of the complexities surrounding cosmetic surgery. However, it highlights the ethical dilemmas the medical profession faced when it tried to decide when and where cosmetic surgery was and was not necessary. In the course of repeated confrontations with exceptional cases, the medical profession was continually forced to go beyond its own discourse and draw upon subjective or commonsense arguments or, more problematically, the available ideological discourses. This meant—at least in the Netherlands—liberal individualism and ethnocentrism.

All attempts to develop general rules for applying guidelines to particular cases failed in the face of myriad exceptions. Medical inspectors for the national health insurance companies openly complained about having to make practical decisions on coverage without having adequate guidelines. And, more seriously, after nearly a decade of trying to get the expansion of cosmetic surgery under control, the number of operations showed no signs of abating.

The medical experts and welfare bureaucrats began to concede that making decisions about who should have cosmetic surgery was a hopelessly subjective enterprise. A short, heated, and somewhat belated public debate ensued. Several plastic surgeons wrote impassioned pieces in the local newspapers defending cosmetic surgery as essential for their patients' well-being. However, these proponents of cosmetic surgery as "welfare surgery" were ultimately overruled. Since the medical profession was unable to back up the welfare argument with a plan for stemming the flow of operations, there was no other recourse but to hand it over to the national health insurance companies. Rather than assessing cosmetic surgery according to the normative criteria recommended by the Dunning Commission, the Council for the National Health Insurance System opted to eliminate cosmetic surgery from the basic health care package.[9] Responsibility for coverage was limited to those few cases that could be justified unproblematically in medical discourse—functional or psychiatric disturbance. The solution to the problem of cosmetic surgery was, therefore, to drop the welfare argument and leave cosmetic surgery for nonfunctional or nonpsychiatric reasons to the private sector.

Recent developments show how short-sighted this ruling was. Since 1991, the number of individuals seeking psychiatric treatment for reasons of appearance has doubled. More than half of all patients contesting decisions concerning national health coverage are applicants for some form of cosmetic surgery. The majority of these appeals are denied and, interestingly, the denial is done in one of two ways. One way is to argue that the applicant's psychological problems are not serious enough to warrant a surgical solution; the other is to claim that the applicant's problems are so extensive that cosmetic surgery will not make a difference. This damned-if-you-do-and-damned-if-you-don't line of reasoning provides a rather chilling indication of the unwillingness on the part of the medical profession and the welfare bureaucrats to take the suffering of cosmetic surgery candidates seriously.

## Back to the Drawing Board

The Dutch case illustrates some of the shortcomings of a discourse of equality, universalism, and distributive justice in the context of a welfare system of health care with limited resources. It shows the drawbacks of an approach that does not place the demand for a particular medical service in the broader social context in which specific groups are differentially involved—either because they express different needs for a medical intervention or because the medical profession is more inclined to dispense certain forms of health care to specific groups. It also shows the limitations of an approach that tries to make choices and cut costs according to general guidelines that are equally applicable to all patients. Applying general rules to individual cases cannot do justice in cases that involve special circumstances or special needs. The Dutch case also shows that the job of cutting costs and making choices cannot and should not be left to the medical profession. It highlights the impossibility of making just choices and defending necessary cutback operations without the participation of patients and other concerned parties.

## *Ethical guidelines*

In *Reshaping the Female Body* (1995), I developed a framework that enabled me to critically situate cosmetic surgery in a broader social, cultural, and political context, while, at the same time, finding a way to justify it as a solution for problems of suffering in special cases. This required a kind of balancing act: finding a way to be critical of the practice which is dangerous, demeaning, or oppressive—without uncritically undermining the women who see it as their best, and, in some cases, only option for alleviating suffering which has gone beyond the point of endurance.

The same balancing act may well be what is required of the medical profession and welfare bureaucracy in their attempts to take seriously the needs of the individual and the limitations of a welfare system where choices in care have to be made. In thinking about ethical guidelines for dealing with controversial medical practices more adequately, I have looked to contemporary feminist ethics for inspiration. Drawing on the work of Iris Young, Nancy Fraser, Seyla Benhabib, and Joan Tronto, an ethical discourse for justifying any medical practices would need to include at least three elements.[10]

First, it would be critical of any argument for or against a particular practice which obscures differences—differences associated with gender, social class, ethnicity or religion, sexual preference, or whatever. Most welfare policy is based on the idea that people are basically the same in terms of their health care needs. However, group differences are often implicated in an individual's bodily experience, sense of well-being, chances of becoming ill, and the kinds of services she or he seeks. It makes no sense to talk about medical interventions like cosmetic surgery as gender-neutral or nonracialized practices. Thus, difference would need to be a starting point for a situated politics of need interpretation.[11]

Second, the ethical guidelines which I envision would have to be critical of any argument that makes it impossible to consider the particularities of the individual case—particularities that are essential for understanding when suffering goes beyond an acceptable limit and intervention is required. Most welfare policy ignores the subjective and local experience of particular individuals and, consequently, tends to turn a blind eye to suffering that falls outside the standard provisions for health care. However, in the interests of minimizing pain that exceeds an acceptable limit, exceptions should be made. For the sake of justice, it may be just as important to know how to make rules as when to break them. Thus, a medical ethics is needed that takes "care" as a moral precept for finding ways to deal with the special case.[12]

Third, an ethics is needed that enables us to be critical of any argument that reduces choices in health care to a matter of distributive justice—that is, to dividing up health care equally among persons who have equal rights to all services. Most welfare policy is not developed in a context of participation and debate and, consequently, does not encourage citizens to take responsibility for the kinds of choices that have to be made in a welfare system. However, a just health care system depends upon its citizens' willingness to support the choices and bear the costs. A feminist ethics of medical care would take solidarity as a point of departure—both in accepting the necessity of making difficult choices as well as in being prepared to shoulder the burden of the special case.[13]

## Conclusion

I have presented a special case in a specific health care system at a specific stage of development. However, as I mentioned at the outset, I believe this case raises a number of questions that have a wider relevance, especially for those who would like to see the U.S. health care system develop in the direction of a welfare model. While it is not my intention to play down the advantages of this model, it behooves us to realize that a welfare system has its difficulties as well, the most notable being that the time invariably comes when everything cannot be done and hard choices need to be made. In that context, questions arise about what constitutes a necessary level of welfare, what should be protected by a basic health care plan, and how health care services can be made available in special cases, when necessary.

Answering these questions requires an ethics that prohibits both a blanket acceptance as well as a straightforward rejection of medical practices and technologies for enhancing the human body. An ethics is needed that can enable us to acknowledge difference, to consider the "exceptional case," and to develop solidarity. Such an ethics would not eliminate the need to make choices in health care. Indeed, it would help us to make them.

## NOTES

1. It has been estimated that more than two million Americans undergo some form of cosmetic surgery every year. See, for example, Naomi Wolf, *The Beauty Myth* (New York: William Morrow, 1991). However, it is virtually impossible to obtain accurate statistics on the actual numbers of operations performed. In both the United States and Europe, statistics are recorded for operations performed in hospitals by registered plastic surgeons. Since the majority of these operations are performed in private clinics and many operations are not performed by plastic surgeons, such estimates do not begin to cover the actual incidence of cosmetic surgery.

2. Even the most minor interventions cause discomfort, ranging from the dead crust of skin left by a chemical peel to the swelling and inflammation of a face-lift. Other operations like abdominoplasties, breast corrections, and liposuctions fall under the category of major surgery, requiring hospitalization and sometimes intensive care. The list of side effects, some permanent, accompanying cosmetic surgery operations is long: infections, wound disruption, scar tissue, pain, numbness, bruising, or discoloration of the skin. More serious disabilities include blood clots, fluid depletion, damage to the immune system, and, in some cases, death. See Kathy Davis, *Reshaping the Female Body: The Dilemma of Cosmetic Surgery* (New York: Routledge, 1995, chapter 1).

3. See, for example, Sandra Bartky, *Femininity and Domination: Studies in the Phenomenology of Oppression* (New York: Routledge, 1990); Iris Marion Young, *Justice and the Politics of Difference* (Princeton: Princeton University Press, 1990); Iris Marion Young, *Throwing Like a Girl and Other Essays in Feminist Philosophy and Social Theory* (Bloomington and Indianapolis: Indiana University Press, 1990); Naomi Wolf, *The Beauty Myth*; Susan Bordo, *Unbearable Weight:*

*Feminism, Western Culture, and the Body* (Berkeley: University of California Press, 1993); Kathy Davis, *Reshaping the Female Body: The Dilemma of Cosmetic Surgery.*

4. The official estimate was 6,060 cosmetic surgery operations between 1980 and 1989, of which 5,925 were women (more than 97 percent). However, since there are 39 private institutes in the Netherlands performing cosmetic surgery, the actual number of operations is considerably higher. National health experts have suggested that 20,000 might be a "modest estimate" though it is nearly four times higher than the official figure!

5. David Frankford. "The Treatment/Enhancement Distinction as an Armament in the Policy Wars," in this volume.

6. The final report was translated into English and used as an example for Hillary Clinton's project to reform the American health care system. See Ministry of Health, Education, and Welfare, *Choices in Health Care* (Rijswijk, the Netherlands: Ministery of Health, Education, and Welfare, 1992).

7. See F. G. Bouman, *De vorm een functie. 25 jaar plastische en reconstructieve chirurgie als specialism in Nederland* (Inaugural Address held at the Faculty of Medicine, Free University, Amsterdam, The Netherlands, 1975).

8. P.M.W. Starmans, "Wat gebeurt er met de esthetische chirurgie?" *Inzet. Opinieblad van de ziekenfondsen,* no. 1 (1988):18–25.

9. Its elimination is surprising, given that cosmetic surgery could easily—and, indeed, effectively—have been assessed according to the four criteria set up by the Dunning Commission.

10. Iris Marion Young, *Justice and the Politics of Difference,* pp. 15–38 and pp. 122–55; Nancy Fraser, *Unruly Practices* (Cambridge: Polity Press, 1987), pp. 161–87; Seyla Benhabib, *Situating the Self: Gender, Community and Postmodernism in Contemporary Ethics* (New York: Routledge, 1992); Joan Tronto, *Moral Boundaries: A Political Argument for an Ethic of Care* (New York: Routledge, 1993)

11. See Nancy Fraser, *Unruly Practices,* and Iris Marion Young, *Justice and the Politics of Difference.*

12. See Seyla Benhabib, *Situating the Self,* and Joan Tronto, *Moral Boundaries.*

13. See Nancy Fraser, *Unruly Practices,* and Iris Marion Young, *Justice and the Politics of Difference,* pp. 15–38.

CAROL FREEDMAN

# Aspirin for the Mind? Some Ethical Worries about Psychopharmacology

In describing the extreme sensitivity to rejection of his patient Lucy, Peter Kramer recounts the following disagreement he had with Sophie Lowenstein Freud.

> Sophie Freud suggested that all people are rejection-sensitive, in the sense that rejection hurts them, but that Lucy might be more skilled than most at *perceiving* rejection. . . .
>
> . . . Sophie Freud's comment . . . is grounded in the belief that all people—if they perceive themselves to be rejected—feel the same pain internally. They differ only according to how small a cue they need to recognize rejection. . . . If all people are similar in how they translate loss into pain, then the instrument we are adjusting is not the internal amplifier but the external receiver—we are asking the person to create an artificial attentional deficit, to ignore loss. . . .
>
> The alternative view—one that seems more likely—is that sensitive people, when they perceive rejection, feel it more keenly. . . . The *primary* deficit is increased amplification. . . .
>
> For the most part, I do not believe that either medicine or psychotherapy makes people less perceptive. But . . . [o]nce we turn down the amplification, small slights, even if they are noticed for a moment, may pass without being registered into memory. . . . In this sense, a *secondary* effect of reduced amplification is reduced perception (emphasis added).[1]

Kramer's disagreement with Sophie Freud might seem to be only an academic quarrel. Kramer argues that when people feel rejected they *first* experience the *pain* of loss, and then the heightened *perception* of loss. Sophie Freud argues, conversely, that what comes first is the heightened *perception* of loss and then the *pain* of loss. They are not disagreeing about the ultimate effect of treatment: for either way the aim is to alter people's perception. They are disagreeing about whether such alteration comes about as a direct or indirect result of treatment. What difference could such a distinction really make?

I want to argue that such a distinction *does* matter. It isn't just a coincidence that Kramer describes his treatment of patients like Lucy as a process of reducing their internal amplifier as opposed to adjusting their external receiver. Analogies in this case have ethical significance. When Kramer discusses the psychological problems he treats with Prozac they are often made to sound like headaches: pains or deficiencies that give rise to particular modes of perception or cognition without being particular modes of perception or cognition themselves. Psychopharmaceuticals, to follow the analogy, are like aspirin.

I want to argue, against the tenor of Kramer's *Listening to Prozac*, that emotional disturbances are often not like headaches, and that once we see this it becomes ethically problematic to treat such disturbances with drugs. Even if we grant, then, that drugs and understanding can realize the same ends of psychic health, the means often make an ethical difference. For what is at stake is a conception of ourselves as responsible agents, not machines.

Central to *Listening to Prozac* is Kramer's claim that Prozac allows us to see a whole spectrum of psychological problems as physical disorders. People who are particularly sensitive to rejection, for example, have problems with their serotonin levels. For the sake of argument, I'll grant Kramer this finding. But I want to challenge some assumptions he makes about what it's like to *experience* emotional problems. In particular, he implies that psychological disturbances are best understood merely as kinds of pain, as is shown in the analogy he makes between rejection-sensitivity and panic disorder.

Panic attacks, he writes, are now understood by psychiatrists as " 'heightened pain in response to loss.' "[2] And this means that the agoraphobia or agrophobia that tend to characterize those who suffer from panic attacks are not *meaningful*. It is not as if one's fear of going over a bridge expressed a terror of being unsupported and insignificant, the way one felt as a small child. For Kramer, "there [is] no special symbolic significance to the bridge, no meaning traceable to childhood trauma or current ambivalence; the only significance of the bridge [is] as an unpleasant place in which to suffer spontaneous panic."[3] Rejection-sensitivity, to follow the analogy, is just a tendency to feel heightened pain in response to loss. And the situations that occasion such pain aren't meaningful.[4]

That Kramer is prone to think of rejection-sensitivity in this way has, I think, less to do with scientific evidence, than with fairly old and unreflective judgments we make at the level of ordinary practice. If Kramer's description of rejection-sensitivity sounds convincing it is more because he is appealing to some common ways we think about the emotions or emotional states,[5] rather than that he is appealing to new developments made possible by ever more sophisticated advances in biological psychiatry.

One common way of thinking about the emotions involves viewing them as noncognitive. What distinguishes an emotion from a cognition, on this view, is a kind of pleasure or pain. These pleasures or pains are influenced by, and influence, cognitions—for example, anger may be caused by the belief that I have been insulted, and it can cause the belief that the offender deserves a piece of my mind. According to this view, emotions are separate from the beliefs that cause them and that they cause. They are not *essentially* connected. It is this sense in which they are like headaches. I do not intend to defend a particular cognitive view of the emotions at length here, but only to raise some questions about the coherence of Kramer's noncognitive account and to examine its ethical implications.[6]

A key question for Kramer's account of emotion is whether it can do justice to the way we *experience* emotion, and in particular to the way in which we see emotion as connected in a *meaningful* way to the situations that cause it. Consider Kramer's case of Lucy. When Lucy was ten her mother was violently murdered. At the time, Lucy showed no immediate reaction. She was productive and responsible, despite the fact that her father focused primarily on his work and not on her. When Lucy first saw Kramer she was a young adult who tended either to become interested in men who were dismissive of her and wild, or to experience heightened feelings of rejection with men who seemed to treat her well. Lucy suffered from deep and protracted moods: "disorganized, paralyzed, hopelessly sad, overtaken by unfocused feelings of urgency."[7] Kramer doesn't deny that we should think of Lucy's current sensitivity to rejection as caused by her past. Even if he thinks of feelings of rejection as nothing more than kinds of pain, he might still think of the places and people Lucy seeks to avoid as meaningful in the sense that they bear a resemblance to the people and places that gave rise to her early experiences of painful rejection. But they are no more meaningful on this view than is my wanting to avoid eating too many hot dogs because eating five once made my stomach upset. Lucy's earliest feelings of rejection on this view were nothing but severe pains occasioned by the murder of her mother. And such early experiences changed Lucy biologically so that she became more prone to feel the pain of rejection. Kramer could argue, then, that because she *associates* such pain with the early experiences that caused it, she seeks to avoid situations that she thinks resemble those early ones.

There are, I think, many problems with understanding the genesis and nature of rejection-sensitivity in this way. But the problem I want to highlight concerns the understanding of emotional states as akin to pleasures or pains that we merely *associate* with types of situations— as if it makes sense to say that Lucy associates the pain of rejection with losing her mother in the way that one might associate a kind of stomach pain with hot dogs. If we reflect carefully about emotional pain, we will realize that the relationship between it and the way we see the situation that we believe causes emotional pain is not like the relationship between physical pain and the way we see the situation that we believe causes physical pain.[8] One notable difference is the fact that emotions are intentional: what I take to be the source of my anger is not separable from the anger itself. There is not my anger, on the one hand, and what I'm angry about on the other. If I am angry about the fact that you are late, then if as I see it you are no longer late, there is no anger. There could be anger about something else. But anger cannot exist without an object in the way that a physical pain can exist without its cause.[9] It is in this sense that emotions are not merely caused by what we take them to be about. And this is why we don't merely *associate* them with what we take them to be about in the way that we might associate hot dogs with stomach pain.

But there is another significant difference between emotions and physical pleasures and pains: the way I see the situation that I believe causes my emotional pain seems from my point of view to *justify* my pain. This notion is revealed by the kinds of reasons we offer for our emotions in contrast to our stomach aches or other physical pains. When we ask someone why their stomach hurts we are in effect asking, "how did it happen that your stomach got upset, what is the *explanation*?" But when we ask Lucy why she feels rejected by her boyfriend, or father, or mother we are not in effect asking, "how did it happen that you came to feel rejected?" We want more than an *explanation*; we want to hear her *justification*. We want to know why Lucy takes feeling rejected to be *merited* by her situation. What sort of evidence does she think there is for believing that certain others don't really care for her?

What as she sees it justifies her level of feeling rejected: what as she sees it merits the view that she is alone in the world, and that no one will ever love her.

Sometimes when we justify our emotions, our reasons terminate in nothing but our own likes and dislikes. When asked, for instance, why I hope there will be vanilla rather than chocolate ice cream at the party, I might respond by saying merely, "because I like vanilla better." But often our reasons for emotions don't terminate in what could be called such "subjectivist" reasons.[10] Why do I feel rejected by the death of my mother? Because it is the worst thing in the world to have no one who sees you standing out in a crowd, who is primarily interested in *your* feelings, achievements, opinions, actions; because I am like an orphan now; I am not whole; there is no one holding me up and watching out for me. And as I feel it, this rejection is not just a matter of how I see things: I am not alone just because I see it that way, and being alone is not bad merely because I don't like it. Being a young girl who feels rejected by the death of her mother is feeling like *the most terrible* thing in the world has happened.

Imagine, then, that when Lucy was a little girl she failed to feel rejected by the murder of her mother. Her failure would be a very different kind of failure from the person who failed to feel a pin prick his finger, or whose knee didn't jump when his reflexes were tested. Both cases reveal problems. The person who doesn't feel the pin prick is not working the way humans usually work; some mechanism is not in normal order. But this explanation does not capture Lucy's problem. For her's is a failure of *insight*—a failure to *see* how really devastating it is to lose the person who has been the center of her world. In this way, emotions are like beliefs. When one feels an inappropriate emotion, it is often like "missing something"—more like a false belief than like failing to feel the prick of the pin or the thump of the hammer. There is a problem, then, with the fact that Kramer thinks of rejection as nothing but a kind of pain, and with rejection-sensitivity as a tendency to feel that pain. Such a view might appeal to our unreflective judgments about the emotions. But such judgments are confirmed neither by scientific evidence, nor by philosophical reflection.[11]

Kramer's account of rejection-sensitivity is unclear because he seems to assume that much of his view follows once we regard a psychological problem as a "quasi-biological quasi-entity."[12] But the fact that a psychological problem is physical does not tell us what it is like for the person having it.[13] We cannot assume that it is merely a kind of pain, that it is like a headache. That this distinction matters ethically when it comes to psychopharmacology is what I want to argue now.

## Insightful Feelings

Psychotherapy in its most basic form carries with it a certain conception of who we are: namely, rational creatures of insight. We can have severely distorted views of the world, and do extremely destructive and inappropriate things. But the psychotherapeutic assumption is that (1) we, often unconsciously, take our distorted and destructive attitudes to be justified; and (2) our justifications, however wrong, are sourced in insight. One of the central goals of psychotherapy is to get the patient to see that she really does take herself to have good reasons for her feelings, and that those reasons originate with insight. This is a deeply respectful and humane aspect of the psychotherapeutic view: our distorted and misguided attitudes are the outgrowth of insightful ones, our craziness the outgrowth of sanity. In Lucy's case, for example, the goal is to get her to see the reasons she takes for her sensitivity to rejection—that is, to get her to see how her conception of herself as deserving rejection is confirmed as she sees it by the fact that her mother abandoned her and her father spent so much time away from home. And this goal is a very small part of the complicated story of justification. The final goal is to get her to see the insight at the heart of her distorted and disturbed view of herself and others: a little girl who really did lose the *central support* of her life, who saw how *utterly irreplacable* such support was.

At the heart of the psychotherapeutic approach is, I think, a view that is indispensible to maintaining the idea of a *self*. To lose a conception of our attitudes as grounded in reasons is to lose a self. If mechanistic causality is the only kind of causality at work in our explanations of why we do and feel what we do, then we are not describing the feelings and behaviors of a self. For central to the idea of a self is the idea of a creature who may legitimately be held responsible. Without a view of ourselves as acting on reasons, we cease to be creatures who may legitimately be held responsible.[14] We become machines. And this means that it is not legitimate for us to ask whether the self may be explainable in mere mechanistic terms, whether it is in fact a machine. For a machine is not a self, and whether there are selves in the world is not a question *for us*. A world without selves is not *our* world. And so, the following sorts of questions must sometimes be answerable in nonmechanistic terms. Why do you think that? Why do you feel that? Why did you do that? The answers, in other words, do not always refer to some physical process: for example, "because my serotonin is too high," "because I'm feeling sick," "because my C-fibers fired in a certain way." Rather, for example: I think abortion is morally permissible *because* I think the fetus is not a person; I feel angry at my friend *because* I think she insulted me; and I came home early *because* I wanted to watch the baseball game on television.[15]

It is important to make one clarification. In what I have said, and will say, I emphasize the essential connection between being a self and acting on reasons, and ultimately rational agency. When many hear this claim, it pushes a button: there is something "off" about seeing ourselves as rational. Surely that's not the right way to describe our emotions. It makes us sound too cool, too calculating. Perhaps I could say instead, "creatures who act on interpretations, self-interpreting animals."[16] But this formulation misses something important, as I see it, that is captured by the idea of acting on reasons. An interpretation is something I don't have to believe is justified, or true. It is not something I have to be committed to. But emotions, for the most part, are our way of being oriented toward what we take to be the true and the good. We might be deeply misguided. But emotions define our characters precisely because they express our deepest beliefs, not just our interpretations. I talk of reasons and rationality, then, with ambivalence. It seems to me that we either lack the language to capture a certain reality, or our conception of reason is so wedded to logic and calculation, as some feminists would argue, that we can only associate the word with certain images.

So being a self means that we will sometimes act, feel, and think for *reasons*. It is important, then, to understand the difference between two types of causality: mechanistic and rational. The therapeutic story about Lucy is an example of rational causality. We take her current way of seeing the world to be one she believes is *justified* by her life and experiences. Her boyfriend turns away every now and then to change the channel on the television, and she feels painfully rejected. As she sees it, when someone's attention to her is distracted she is being *ignored*. Being ignored is not being cared for; it is not a far cry away from being abandoned. Such a way of interpreting things is justified as Lucy sees it because that is what experience has shown her—for example, her father's constant turning away from her at a time in her life when she already felt lost and alone. Her conception of herself as ignored and not cared for is rationally caused in the sense that it is something she believes to be grounded in good reasons.

A headache, on the other hand, is an example of mechanistic causation. I might have a headache that is caused by psychological stress—my bank account is running low, I'm late on the rent, or my child has the flu. In this sense my headache is caused by my interpretations: I believe I am not succeeding in supporting and caring for my child properly, and am, therefore, a bad parent. These are interpretations I take myself to be justified in having. We could say, then, that the beliefs that give rise to my headache are rationally caused. But this doesn't mean the headache is so caused. For the relationship between the headache and my interpretations is mechanistic: I don't take my headache to be *justified* by the way I see the world. My headache is not something I take to be grounded in good reason. Rather it is the *result* of a way of seeing the world that I take myself to have good reasons for.[17]

In making a distinction between two kinds of causality the point is not to deny the intimate connection between our interpretations and our embodiment. The point is not to be a dualist: as if there were pure mind and pure body. The point is that we are dehumanized if we are reduced to mere mechanism. And that means that we must distinguish between those actions and attitudes that we are going to regard as interpretative and those that we are going to regard as physical.

For Kramer, feeling rejected is like having a bad headache, and suffering from rejection-sensitivity is like being prone to suffer from a bad headache. To see Lucy's problem as unconnected to her self-interpretations, as a problem of "internal amplification," is to see it as mechanistically caused. It is like a headache in the sense that it might be caused by self-interpretations that are themselves rationally caused. So a by-product of Lucy's view of herself as undeserving of love may be the feeling of, and proneness to feeling, rejection. And her feeling of rejection might cause a change in her self-interpretations. But the relationship between the self-interpretations that both cause, and are caused by, the feeling of rejection is mechanistic. The feeling of rejection is, like a headache, just a kind of pain. And in this sense, it is typically not something one takes oneself to have *reason* to feel.

I would like to propose that seeing our psychological problems as like headaches has the following ethical implications. Crudely put, you could think of psychological problems as existing on a spectrum. At one extreme are problems that are clearly untreatable by insight and understanding. At the other end of the spectrum are problems whose prospects for being treatable by insight and understanding are not so clear. When it comes to the ethical appropriateness of treating psychological problems with drugs there is, in one sense, only one relevant question: *can* the problem be treated with insight or understanding? If we judge the problem to be one that only responds to physical intervention, then that seems to be sufficient for determining that drug use is ethically appropriate. But it doesn't mean that if we judge that the problem *can* be treated with drugs, then it is ethically appropriate to do so. It is here the headache analogy becomes relevant. If you are suffering from a headache, then whether it is ethically appropriate for you to take aspirin doesn't seem to hang on whether drugs are the only way to remove your discomfort. We might believe that thinking good thoughts while sitting in the bathtub could relieve your pain, but that seems to have no bearing on whether it is ethically appropriate for you to take an aspirin. You have a headache. It is painful. Aspirin will help. That is all there is to it.

That we have this ethical judgment about headaches is grounded, I think, in the fact that they are mechanistically caused. Emotional problems, I've suggested, can be like suffering from false beliefs.[18] Lucy, for example, is *wrong* to see herself as ignored and abandoned by her boyfriend just because he changes the channel on the television. And her false beliefs, we can imagine, are grounded in something like a *mistake in reasoning*. So Lucy might be right to see her father's treatment of her as a case of being ignored and abandoned. But she is mistaken to believe further that when others fail to pay her undivided attention *they* don't care for her, and that she is undeserving of the love of a good person. When we see someone's problem as a mistake in reasoning, there is an imperative to help them understand their error. For that is the way we value our capacity as creatures who act on reasons. Valuing the fact that we act on reasons means trying to correct mistakes in reasoning with other reasons.[19] To think it is appropriate to "cure" mistakes of reasons mechanistically is to regard our rational capacity as of little significance or importance. That—insofar as we live in a world of selves—is something we are in no position to do. It is in this sense that it matters what means we use to 'cure' our psychological problems.[20]

To know that a psychological problem responds to drugs, then, is not sufficient for determining that such treatment is ethically appropriate. We will want to know how the problem is caused—mechanistically or rationally. And that is not answered for us merely by knowing that the problem is physical and that it responds to drugs. There will certainly be considerable variation among those psychological problems that might be resolvable with insight and understanding: there will be those problems that are better addressed with psychotherapy and those that are not; those problems that require long-term psychotherapy and those that do not. These will be tough cases ethically. Even if we judge our problems to be rationally caused by our self-interpretations, they might still respond to drugs. Then we will have to consider our reservations about taking drugs in light of the following questions. How long in therapy is too long? Does treating the problem with drugs facilitate therapy, and in that sense is it in the service of insight and understanding? With cases at this end of the spectrum, however, it will be clear that once we see our problem as rationally caused our objective should be insight and understanding. So drug use in these cases ought always to be in the service of insight and understanding, and there should always be a healthy resistance to drugs.[21] For many emotional problems are precisely not like headaches. They are not *just* painful. And so, even if drugs work, that's not all there is to it.[22]

The headache analogy reveals how important it is for us to describe the problems we treat with drugs as problems *of the body*—problems that can no doubt *affect* the mind without themselves being "of the mind." We aren't troubled by the way vitamins affect our minds, for example, because we think of ourselves as attending to the body so that the mind can "do its thing." Treating our emotional problems with drugs might sometimes be like taking vitamins or fixing low blood sugar. But if we think of all emotional problems as mechanical problems, we lose our personhood. It is too easy, and dangerous to think of all psychopharmacological drugs as like aspirin, or vitamins.

What is particularly interesting about the headache analogy is the extent to which it appeals to ordinary experience. Scientists can tell you that your problem is "of the body," and mean that it is your hormones, or your serotonin, or something similar. But a headache is "of the body" at the level of felt experience; it is a pain. We define it as bodily, as mechanistically caused, in our *own* understanding of it. The task of determining causation is infinitely complicated. Whether biological psychiatry can definitively show that a psychological problem is caused by a physical problem, as opposed to merely being physically realized, is questionable.[23] It is no wonder, then, that Kramer appeals to something like the headache analogy. It seems to make his way of describing emotional problems more persuasive. For we as ordinary people can appreciate the extent to which emotional problems are bodily. They seem to be like pains. I'm afraid that this is how our culture is being encouraged to think about emotional problems by the current revolution in biological psychiatry. What I have argued, however, is that our unreflective understanding of emotion is mistaken. Much of the appeal of Kramer's analogy, then, is in the end ungrounded.

## Conclusion

My argument can be summarized as follows.

(1) The familiar view that emotions are merely kinds of pleasures and pains is not something science can show. To describe the physiology of a psychological state doesn't tell us what it is like to experience such a state and, in this respect, doesn't inform us as to what an emotion is.

(2) On my view, emotions are not merely like pains that are caused by and cause beliefs, interpretations, and perceptions. Emotions, unlike headaches, are themselves ways of believing and interpreting, even though they are physically realized and viscerally felt.

(3) When an emotional problem is sourced in our interpretations or reasons, then we should have a basic commitment to addressing it with insight and understanding. Otherwise, we are not respecting what it is to be a self. For central to maintaining the idea of a self is the commitment to regard some of our actions and attitudes as justified by our reasons, not explained in mechanistic terms. My view concedes that the treatment of some emotional problems that are sourced in our reasons may be facilitated by medication. But even in such cases there should be a healthy resistance to drugs.[24]

(4) The current revolution in biological psychiatry—as interpreted in Peter Kramer's *Listening to Prozac*—encourages us to think of emotional problems as like headaches. This is a convenient view, for if we can say that what someone is *experiencing* is just pain, then there is little doubt that her problem should be regarded in mechanistic terms. We don't need a scientist to tell us the physiology of headaches to believe that it is appropriate to treat headaches with aspirin.

(5) Kramer's view is troubling, then, because it makes it too easy for us to see ourselves in mechanistic terms. In this sense it jeopardizes our dignity as responsible persons who owe it to ourselves to struggle toward insight through dialogue.[25]

## NOTES

**1.** Peter Kramer, *Listening to Prozac* (New York: Penguin Books, 1993), pp. 103–04.

**2.** Kramer, *Listening to Prozac*, p. 77.

**3.** Kramer, *Listening to Prozac*, p. 82.

**4.** Kramer's general tendency to see emotional problems as meaningless is evident in the way he contrasts his view with psychoanalysis. See, especially, *Listening to Prozac,* chapter 4.

**5.** Though Kramer describes rejection-sensitivity as a disorder of *mood*, it is still appropriate to talk here of his view of emotion. For while rejection-sensitivity is not described as an emotion per se, it is described as an affective, as distinct from a cognitive, problem. It seems in this sense to be essentially emotional in nature.

In the chapter on self-esteem, for example, Kramer says explicitly that medication treats affective, as distinct from cognitive, problems. He emphasizes a number of times throughout the chapter that self-esteem, insofar as it is an affective condition, is not primarily a matter of self-understanding. Self-esteem can *influence* self-understanding, but not the other way around. See, especially, pp. 208–12, 221.

**6.** The contemporary philosophical literature on the emotions is dominated by attempts of one form or another to defend a cognitive view of the emotions. See, for example: Robert Roberts, "What an Emotion Is: A Sketch," *Philosophical Review*, Vol. 97, n. 2 (1988); Cheshire Calhoun, "Cognitive Emotions?" in *What is an Emotion?* ed. Cheshire Calhoun and Robert Solomon (New York: Oxford University Press, 1984), pp. 327–42; Amelie Oksenberg Rorty, "Explaining Emotions," in *Explaining Emotions*, ed. Amelie Oksenberg Rorty (Berkeley: University of California Press, 1980), pp. 103–26; Ronald de Sousa, *The Rationality of Emotion* (Cambridge: MIT Press, 1987); Patricia Greenspan, *Emotions and Reasons* (New York: Routledge, 1988); Anthony Kenny, *Action, Emotion and Will* (New York: Humanities Press, 1964); and Irving Thalberg, *Perception, Emotion and Action* (New Haven: Yale University Press, 1977).

**7.** Kramer, *Listening to Prozac*, p. 69.

**8.** One could argue that emotions are pains or pleasures that we associate with cognitions in an *essential*, rather than contingent, way. We could call such a view a "causal cognitive" account. For according to such a view emotion would not be a pain or pleasure that is associated with cognition *in the way* that physical pains are associated with cognitions. And so, emotions would not be, to make a familiar philosophical argument, like *sensations*. Kramer, however, views emotions as akin to sensations. In criticizing his view, then, I am not criticizing a "causal cognitive" view, but a view of emotion as akin to sensation.

The "causal cognitive" view, for the most part, captures the basic structure of Hume's account of the "indirect passions"—even though Hume himself is not always Humean. See, in particular, his discussion of pride in *The Treatise*, ed. L.A. Selby-Bigge and P.H. Niditch (New York: Oxford University Press, 1990), pp. 275–89. Others who often sound like endorsers of the causal cognitive view include Robert Gordon, *The Structure of Emotions* (Cambridge: Cambridge University Press, 1987). For a reading of Gordon that makes his view look causal, see Robert Roberts's review in *Philosophical Review*, Vol. 99, No. 2 (1990). Freud explicitly endorses what could be called a weak version of the "causal cognitive" view—where emotion tends to be associated with beliefs of a certain sort, though the two can be separated. But Freud misdescribes his own insights here. That his explicit theory of emotion often fails to do justice to the practice of psychoanalysis is argued quite persuasively by Jonathan Lear in *Love and Its Place in Nature* (New York: Farrar, Straus and Giroux, 1990), pp. 91–93.

**9.** For some classic discussions of the nature of emotional causes and objects, see Irving Thalberg, *Perception, Emotion and Action*, excerpted in Calhoun and Solomon, *What is an Emotion?* pp. 291–304; Anthony Kenny, *Action, Emotion and Will*, excerpted in Calhoun and Solomon, *What is an Emotion?* pp. 279–90; and Robert Solomon, "Emotions and Choice," also excerpted in Calhoun and Solomon, *What is an Emotion?*

**10.** The distinction between "subjectivist" and "objectivist" reasons is one way of capturing Charles Taylor's distinction between "weak" and "strong" evaluation. See his, "What is Human Agency?" in *Philosophical Papers I*, (Cambridge: Cambridge University Press, 1985), pp. 15–44.

**11.** I am not denying that *some* psychological disturbances might be nothing but kinds of pain. The main problem with Kramer's account is that he wants to entertain the possibility that all emotional disorders should be conceived on the model of rejection-sensitivity—this is what we are led to believe, he suggests, when we "listen to Prozac." What I am challenging, then, is the view that Kramer is accurately giving us anything like the model of emotional disturbance.

**12.** Kramer, *Listening to Prozac*, p. 105.

**13.** To talk about what a mental state "is like" is, for many, another way of talking about the subjective irreducibility of mental states. See, for example, Thomas Nagel's "What Is It Like to Be a Bat?" in *Mortal Questions* (Cambridge: Cambridge University Press, 1979), pp. 165–80. When I use the phrase, "what it is like . . . ," however, I am not making any claims about the subjective irreducibility of mental states. I am just questioning whether the activity of describing the biological nature of mental states can adequately determine whether such states are, for example, pains, desires, or beliefs.

**14.** That we cannot deny the truth of the perspective from which we are responsible agents is argued by, among others, Thomas Nagel in "Moral

Luck," in *Mortal Questions*, pp. 24–38, and Peter Strawson in "Freedom and Resentment," *Proceedings of the British Academy*, vol. 48 (1962), pp. 1–25.

That responsible agency requires acting on reasons is essentially uncontroversial in the contemporary philosophical literature on the topic. *What* counts as acting on a reason, however, and *why* responsible agency requires acting on a reason are questions that motivate much disagreement. For some well-known discussions, see Donald Davidson, "Actions, Reasons and Causes," in *Actions and Events* (New York: Oxford University Press, 1989), pp. 3–20; Harry Frankfurt, "Freedom of the Will and the Concept of a Person," in *The Importance of What We Care About* (New York: Cambridge University Press, 1988), pp. 11–25; Charles Taylor, "What Is Human Agency?" and Susan Wolf, "Sanity and the Metaphysics of Responsibility," in *Responsibility, Character, and the Emotions,* ed. Ferdinand Schoeman (New York: Cambridge University Press, 1987), pp. 46–62. For a nice summary of different stories of how human action originates, see David Velleman, "The Guise of the Good," *Nous* 26:1 (1992), pp. 3–5.

**15.** To describe a case of causation as rational is compatible with "the body's" playing a role in two senses. First, insofar as we are embodied creatures, it will always be the case that we depend upon the body's functioning in order for our rational processes to operate. It is assumed, then, that when a rational explanation holds, certain mechanistic processes are required as well. We all need sleep and proper nutrition, for example. But insofar as the self requires a domain of rational explanation, there must be some legitimate distinction between the kind of minimal role the body plays in cases of rational causation, as compared to the significant role it plays in cases of mechanistic causation.

Second, to say that the self requires cases of rational causation does not preclude there also being mechanistic explanations for the same cases. So for any instance when an explanation in terms of an agent's reasons holds, there might *also* be a physical explanation that holds as well. I can accurately describe my walking in the house and turning on the television both as, "I came home because I wanted to watch the ballgame," and "my C-fibers caused my muscles to move." There might be two levels of explanation in this sense. That is why understanding mental phenomena in physical terms does not settle whether there is also a rational account to be told. All that the self requires is that a rational explanation sometimes be true.

**16.** The expression, "self-interpreting animals" comes from Charles Taylor's essay "Self-interpreting Animals," in *Philosophical Papers 1*, pp. 45–76.

**17.** This is not to say that one's headache could not be rationally caused. I could make it my objective to have a headache. I might unconsciously see having physical pain as something there is good reason to have—perhaps to get my husband's sympathy, or because I believe I am a bad parent and I deserve to suffer discomfort. But this is not the typical case. In the typical case my headache is the by-product of attitudes that I take myself to be justified in having. Usually the attitudes are rationally caused; the headache is not.

**18.** One of the complicated implications of thinking of emotions as like beliefs is that it is not clear how we are to treat someone who is experiencing painful, but *justified* emotion. If it were always, and simply, the case that seeing the truth helped an agent—by perhaps motivating action in the long run that protects her from harm—then feeling justified emotion should always be encouraged. But since it is not clear that the truth always benefits an agent, we will sometimes have to weigh our commitment to reducing suffering against our commitment to grasping the truth.

**19.** It might be objected that even if we grant that understanding matters, it doesn't follow that such understanding must be achieved through insight. As a compatibilist might argue, all that matters is that we are creatures who act on reasons, it doesn't matter how we got to be such creatures. Suffice it to say, however, that I am assuming a compatibilism of a Strawsonian sort. On the one hand, whether determinism is true doesn't matter when it comes to our status as responsible agents. On the other hand, from within the practical standpoint, it is as if determinism is false. I am interested in showing what follows from within the practical standpoint. And that means that if it matters that I get from point a to point b by rational means, than it also matters that I get to point a by rational means.

**20.** There are at least two other important arguments for why the means matter when it comes to treating psychological problems: one has to do with the kind of good that character is, and the other has to do with the importance of suffering. While I don't have the space here to look at such arguments in depth, it is worth mentioning how my argument supplements and corrects these arguments in important ways.

So, for example, when articulating why character is the kind of thing that ought to be achieved in certain ways, it is not enough merely to say it is valued as the product of our will. For there are many things that we may be responsible for—like a stress headache—that we don't think it is wrong to treat with drugs. It is because character is the product of our will in the sense that it is sourced in *our reasons*, then, that explains why it should not be achieved primarily in mechanistic ways. And it is not enough to say that character is the kind of good that is valued as the product of effort and discipline. For what matters is that character be changed as a result of a certain *kind* of effort and discipline: the kind that follows, among other things, from the fact that character is sourced in reasons.

The argument that there is intrinsic value in suffering, that it has value apart from the ends it promotes, is also supplemented by my argument. For it is difficult to imagine how suffering could have such intrinsic value if it were *just pain*; that is, if it involved no insight, if it were not cognitive. And so, my argument is a way of explaining why insight as a means to psychic health matters.

**21.** But what are we to say about someone who has important commitments—like finishing his novel—who doesn't want to spend the time it would take to change himself through understanding? I would argue that while someone like this has good reason to take drugs for his emotional problems, there is always a kind of *loss* involved in not choosing to pursue understanding as the preferable way of correcting problems that are sourced in our reasons. Ethical life is not just about seeking to minimize pain. It involves evaluating a variety of goods, and making tough choices. Sometimes the goods we choose between are incommensurable, and we are left "missing out" on something valuable even when our choices are justified. But the basic commitment to correct problems that are sourced in our reasons through understanding is a good of such fundamental value to us as rational agents, that to fail to make it a priority involves a fundamental loss. It might sometimes be justified. But doing the right thing in such a case should still leave us with some reluctance and ambivalence.

**22.** Once we recognize that many emotional problems are not just painful, it follows that the purpose of psychotherapy is not just to relieve suffering. It will often be a *primary* goal of psychotherapy to change perception. And this raises difficult questions about the conception of therapy as *health care*. Suffice it to say that I don't think it is in the interest of psychotherapy to misdescribe what it does in the attempt to gain credibility and funding.

**23.** For an excellent discussion of the limits of biological psychiatry's ability to mark out the causes of mental illness, see Colin A. Ross and Alvin Pam, *Pseudoscience in Biological Psychiatry* (New York: John Wiley and Sons, 1995).

**24.** Having a healthy resistance to psychopharmacology does not mean believing that anyone should be coerced into having therapy or denied access to safe medication. It does mean, however, believing that psychotherapy should be treated as a legitimate form of treatment, and that people should be provided with a real opportunity to get it—something that is beginning to sound radical in our present age of managed-care.

**25.** I am indebted for criticism to Michael Della Rocca, Jodi Halpern, Carol Rovane, Lawrence Vogel, members of the "enhancement technologies" project at the Hastings Center, and audiences at Connecticut College and Worcester Polytechnic Institute.

RONALD COLE-TURNER

# Do Means Matter?

New technology often gives us new ways to do something we have always done, or at least always wished we could do. And new technology is often accepted as good or moral because it helps us achieve established ends more easily or efficiently. In medicine, for instance, new techniques such as noninvasive surgery are quickly accepted because they achieve the same ends as the older techniques, and in fact do so with certain advantages. And in ethics, one sometimes hears an argument of this form: The new technique is acceptable because, after all, we have always achieved the same end through another means.

But what if the end in view is something like improved classroom performance by grade school children? This end can be achieved through reduced class size (using traditional or established means) or through prescriptions for Ritalin for some of the students (a new means). If the traditional ends and means are good, is the new means also good? Does using Ritalin instead of reducing class size to achieve this end make a moral difference?

Or what if the end is heightened cognitive performance, which can be achieved through classic educational strategies, but which some day in the future might be achievable by genetic techniques, possibly even by human germ-line genetic enhancement. Again we might wonder: If the traditional ends and means are good, is the futuristic means? Would using genetics instead of education to achieve this end make a morally significant difference in the meaning of the end?

Some, of course, will argue that psychopharmacology or genetic alteration may affect the body or the brain but not the person as person, not the soul or the mind, not the self as a psychological dimension of being.[1] In this view, pills can never replace education, nor can genetics ever affect the essential self. This view is based on some form of dualism of brain and mind or of body and soul and is probably very widespread, even if its religious or philosophical antecedents have disappeared. It provides a certain reassurance, to those who hold it, that technology has its limits, confined to the body and incapable of touching the soul, and so technology simply cannot replace certain traditional means, such as education, meditation, or other personal or mental disciplines. The dualism on which this objection is based is, of course, under attack, and the reasons given are often found in the very science and technology that cause us to ask these questions in the first place. Psychopharmacology—Prozac, in particular—seems to many to affect the essential self, the soul, in much the same ways as traditional religious activities.[2]

As we learn more about the brain, we learn that mental activity has neuroanatomical consequences, that the brain itself is shaped by its use. For instance, the brains of the players of stringed instruments are anatomically different from the brains of the rest of us.[3] A traditional discipline—playing the violin, or perhaps reading Shakespeare or praying—if practiced over a significant period of time, affects the very structure of the brain. Now if, some day in the distant future, the structural effect could be achieved, not through discipline but through technology, would the full effect be the same? I will return to this question in the final section of this essay; for now, however, I want to point out that as support for anthropological dualism erodes, the question of technological vs. traditional means is laid bare.

The question of means is raised by the emergence of the technologies of enhancement. But before we consider the significance of means in seeking certain human enhancements, we should note that the question of means can also arise in relation to therapy or treatment. In 1997 in western Pennsylvania, the state found a couple guilty of involuntary manslaughter in the death of their sixteen-year-old daughter, who died of complications of diabetes because they did not seek medical help, choosing instead to pray for her. If they had sought medical help and she still died, it is not very likely that they or the hospital or medical staff would have been indicted. That the parents failed in restoring health to their daughter seems less important to the case than that they chose the wrong means, at least in the view of the state and of most people. While few would support the choice of these parents, it is fair to note that there is growing interest in the relationship between spiritual and other alternative forms of healing, and so we should expect that questions about the means of therapy will become more urgent and more confusing. How do we agree on the best means, on acceptable means, and on unacceptable means for treatment?

When we turn to the prospect of medical or scientific means of human enhancement, the question of means becomes all the more difficult. The reason is not that we in Western culture are against enhancement, or that our philosophical or religious traditions warn us against it, while technology seems to offer a new temptation. It is rather that we in Western culture are enhancement enthusiasts.

For example, in Christianity, personal enhancement is the central organizing motif: Human beings are redeemed (some would say "born again") into a new mode of existence. And virtually everyone in the West agrees on the importance of education or on other forms of human effort in pursuit of one's goals. Life for us is one long project of self-improvement. So it is hardly the case that technology offers enhancement while Western religion or philosophy defends the human status quo. On the contrary, technology is worrisome precisely because it offers a new means to achieve the old ends. Technologies such as psychopharmacology and human genetic manipulation fit very well within the broad program of Western religions and philosophy.

But therein lies the problem. For when we ask about the ethics of a new technology of human enhancement, we can readily imagine this argument being made: We have, after all, always sought to achieve these goals through traditional means; the new means seek the same goals, but they achieve them more quickly or efficiently; therefore, the new means are good, perhaps even better than the old means.

The prospect of hearing this argument, especially when applied to psychopharmacology or to genetics, immediately gives rise to a worry, at least for some, that we are missing something important and that we are sliding too easily from old means to new, without looking carefully for the moral difference between them. We find ourselves worrying that such an argument is destined more to obscure than to illuminate, more to blind that to examine. "We have always done this by other means" may be comforting, but is it sound moral reasoning? Or so the worry asks.

## Two Arguments and Their Limits

What lies behind this worry? Does it point to an important intuition about new means and their relationship to old means and old ends, or is it merely a form of nostalgia or technophobia? In order to unfold this concern more fully, two arguments have been suggested. First, it is sometimes thought that old means are in some sense natural, while new means are artificial. The objection here is not the naive claim that nature is always good and artifice bad, or that by "nature" we mean "traditional," which is good, while by "artificial" we really mean "nontraditional," which is bad. The objection may be more forcefully stated in this way: It is natural to human beings to nourish and indeed to enhance themselves and their children by means of good diet, education, moral example, or religious activity. Parents who do these things for their children are to be praised for doing what human parents naturally should do. Furthermore (and more important), these activities are not so much means to an end—such as enhancing our children or equipping them to get ahead in a competitive world—as they are the natural expression of parental affection. As such, they are never simply replaceable by other means, which might include anything such as vitamin pills, music lessons, special sports instruction, or psychopharmacology. It is not that any of these other means are necessarily bad or inappropriate in the right situations; they are just not the sorts of things that human parents are naturally expected to do for their children, or that human beings are naturally expected to do for themselves.

While this argument has serious limitations if seen as an argument against unnatural or artificial means, it does point to an important insight, namely, that not everything we do is a means to an end. Some things are done simply out of self-respect, or out of love for another, or out of a sense of what is appropriate in a relationship, such as that between parent and child. A mother does not hug her newborn in order to enhance its future emotional and cognitive state, although we now know that this will occur as a result of her action. She hugs her infant for the sake of love and joy, not as a means to an end. So to suggest that some future pill might accomplish the same end is to commit a category mistake. A pill is not therefore bad; it simply occupies a different moral space, and its legitimacy needs to be argued on other grounds than by saying that it achieves the same thing as a mother's hug.

For people of religious conviction and practice, the observance of the rituals of a tradition are not so much means to an end. Observing one's faith may make one feel "closer to God," or it might even improve one's health by helping to relieve stress or by providing systems of social support. But religious people do not follow the practices of their faith *in order to* achieve these ends; rather, they do them because they believe that they live in such a universe, or in the presence of such a God, that worship is the natural or fitting response. People worship, not because it gets much accomplished, but because if there is a God, it is the right thing to do. Once again, some future pill might accomplish the same effects as religious practice; but to suggest that it achieves the same ends as religion is to misunderstand religion, for the practice of religion is not about achieving ends but about a right relationship with that which is ultimate.

Now of course, as culture and technology change, "what parents naturally do for their children" or "what people naturally do for themselves" also changes. We today regard it as a fairly natural thing for parents to read books to their children by incandescent light, something which could not be done before light bulbs or, for most people by any light, before the printing press. The argument's value is not in helping us decide whether new means are right or wrong but in confronting us with the instrumentalism that characterizes so much of our thinking. Not everything we do is a means to an end.

The second argument is this: Assume that new means are effective in achieving traditional ends, such as athletic or intellectual accomplishment. The new means, such as psychopharmacology and genetic alteration, are perhaps more efficient or easier than the traditional means.[4] But for that reason, they should be opposed, because there is value in the traditional means themselves, quite independent of the ends they achieve. By offering us an easy way to achieve the end, the new means cheat us of the value to be found in the old means. There is, after all, a glory and a dignity in human accomplishment attained the "old-fashioned way," through sweat and struggle, sometimes against great odds. It is something like the mountain climber who struggles to the top of a great peak, but then on flying home ascends quickly by jet over the top of the mountain, and looking down at the summit, feels cheated of the value of the original climb. Technology, precisely because of its power and efficiency, seems to cheat us of the experience of accomplishment, which is something valued in distinction from the achievement of the end.

The significance of this argument lies in its calling attention to the value that lies in certain means, over and above the value found in the end considered by itself. The value in climbing the mountain peak— the physical and mental discipline, the experience of the gradually opening vistas, the sense of personal accomplishment—are all distinct from the value of being at the summit. Attaining the summit by a new, technological means might be a good thing under some circumstances, but if the new technical possibility generally discouraged people from attempting the old means, the extra value that lay distinctly in the old means would be lost. Indeed, there may be some areas of human activity in which the value that is distinctive to the means far exceeds the value found in achieving the end. Mountain climbers are likely to claim this argument for their sport. If it is correct, then a new means will be a poor trade-off. It is not so much that people would be cheated by technology but that they would be tempted to cheat themselves through technology. This argument, by calling attention to what we might lose, warns us of the cost of cheating.

This argument should not, however, be taken as an objection to the use of new means, for the simple reason that while new means may relocate our human struggle, they do not eliminate it. The fact that I write at a computer makes writing easier by eliminating retyping and other frustrations, but writing itself is an intense struggle, and it will remain so under any technological condition. The technological advance does not eliminate the struggle so much as relocate it; indeed, it makes it possible to eliminate secondary aggravations and focus attention on the core struggle at hand, namely, expressing new insight in just the right words. Even if technology increased our cognitive ability itself, not just by giving us faster computers but faster brains, so that we could calculate or write or think more clearly, these activities would still be a struggle in the face of even greater intellectual challenges to which we human beings would inevitably set ourselves. Therefore, any concern that new, technological means eliminates human struggle altogether seems ill-founded; and thus, this argument should not be taken as a categorical objection to the use of new, technological means to achieve ends formerly achieved through other means. At the same time, it offers an important warning, namely, that we should consider carefully the value that is distinctive to the old means, value that could be lost if we simply replace old means with new.

## Ends and Other Effects

In this final section, I want to return to the question of dualism and its demise and to explore further how our anthropology (or conception of the human) becomes a factor in this discussion. To me, at least, it is distressing that precisely at the moment in human history when we are poised on the threshold of the possibility of the technological manipulation of human nature, we have very little consensus on what we mean by human nature. In fact, we have very few candidate theories of human nature, philosophical or theological, and so it is quite likely we will proceed to alter what we do not even pretend to understand. It may turn out that through our self-alteration, through a kind of scientific experiment on ourselves, we will come at last to understand ourselves more clearly.

A strong anthropological dualism would permit us to say that there are physical and technological means that affect the body and even the brain, but that there are also social, psychological, intellectual, and spiritual means that affect the self or the soul, and that these two categories do not compete or overlap with each other. Any amount of future technological alteration of the brain would leave human beings in roughly the same social and spiritual predicament in which we currently find ourselves.

If we reject such dualism, we will recognize that already with psychopharmacology, and in the future with genetics, it will be possible to alter the brain in ways that alter the self or the soul. If so, then these questions quickly arise: Is the alteration of the self by technical means the same as its alteration by traditional means? Is there a morally significant difference between different means and their effects? If so, can an analysis of this difference offer us any guidance in making decisions about the proper use of new technologies, particularly in respect to questions of social justice?

I want to consider each of these questions. First, is the alteration of the self by technical means the same as its alteration by traditional means? I will argue that it is not. Now if we define what we mean by "alteration" narrowly, as a specific, measurable end, it may be possible to achieve the same end through technology as through traditional means. But if we agree to such a narrow definition, we will have already made an important decision about the relationship between a specific end to be achieved and the full range of effects that result from our use of one means as opposed to another. That decision, to focus on a narrow definition of an end, is consistent with a broad tendency of modern thought toward that which is specific, measurable, abstracted from its full context of meaning, and therefore "thin." This tendency of thought contains a built-in prejudice for technology, for by defining ends narrowly, it allows us to think that technology achieves them.

The alternative to such "thin" description is not dualism but the recognition of the essential "thickness" of human experience, even when it is described strictly at the genetic/neurological level. For instance, in saying that a pill achieves the same effect as prayer, we might mean that the pill makes us feel the same way, or that it brings the level of serotonin or other key neurotransmitters to the same parameters as does prayer. We can criticize this claim at its psychological level: Prayer and the pill do not really make us feel the same way, for even if the effects are experienced as the same *in some respects* (relaxation, confidence, self-assurance), in other respects (an awareness of the obligations imposed by God, for example), they are hardly the same. But we can also criticize this claim at the molecular and cellular level: Prayer and the pill do not really achieve the same neurological effects, for even if the serotonin level looks the same, prayer is a robust mental activity with countless other neurological correlates, all occurring in a markedly different sequence of neural events, from the effects of a pill.

Now of course, we could persist in the tendency of modern thought and choose a narrow or "thin" account of change and point to how the two means attain the same end. But doing so prejudices the matter in favor of technology in particular and substitute means in general. Any means, any human activity, has a rich array of effects, some of which we are aware, some of which we are not, some of which are intended, and some of which may be regretted. When we consider the full array of effects, we see that significantly different means can (and often do) have significantly different effects.

So then we ask: Is there a morally significant difference between different means and their effects? To which, of course, I would answer yes. The weight of the significance will depend on the person making the decision between alternative means. For example, if we want to be less anxious and more self-confident and we believe this state can be attained either through prayer or through a pill, our choice will depend on whether there are other effects, contingent upon either one of these means, that are either to be desired or avoided. If we simply want to be relieved of anxiety quickly, the pill is the obvious choice. If we believe there are manifold effects of prayer, and we value them, we might choose prayer. My point here is not that one choice is right and the other wrong; that depends on the broader matrix of values to which a person adheres. My point is simply that different means bring about different effects that may be morally significant.

Which leads us to ask: Can an analysis of this difference offer us any guidance in making decisions about the proper use of new technologies, particularly in respect to social justice? If we are looking here for general guidance, I think the answer is no. As we make our way into the era of human technological self-transformation, we will no doubt find ourselves learning as we go. In this sense, we may discover who we are by changing what we are—a risky enterprise, to be sure, but from all indications our most likely course.

As a society, we should hope that we will learn from each other how new means mix with old, whether they conflict or complement each other, and where the general warnings or dangers might lie. For instance, there is a growing concern that psychopharmacology is being used, not for therapy or even for enhancement in the sense of self-development, but as a booster to equip us for an increasingly competitive society. One can imagine the temptation to use genetics in the same way, to give our offspring an advantage against their enhanced competitors. But when we think honestly about this, we begin to wonder if we have not already used education in precisely the same way, to give a privileged advantage to some of our offspring so that they may outperform those not so advantaged. If in fact we have used traditional means unjustly, we need to be particularly wary that new means will fall under the familiar patterns of injustice, perhaps augmenting their magnitude. These questions are further complicated by the differences among human beings and by our increased reliance upon technology to mitigate or to remove these differences. If genetics is the science of differences, will human genetic engineering become the technology of their removal? And if so, will we see this as good or bad?

The new technological means of human alteration offered by psychopharmacology and genetics will present new challenges to social justice, for they could alternatively be used to remove or to expand human differences. What are we to make (literally and figuratively) of those who differ from the rest of us? Suppose someone wants to be religious but cannot do so without the aid of psychopharmacology. Others of us, probably the overwhelming majority, can be religious without this form of help, although we may require other forms. Indeed, for most strands of the Christian tradition, *all* people need help in the form of divine grace if they are to be religious. But what then are we to think of those individuals who seem to need psychopharmacology in addition to other means of help? Or what are we to make of those individual school children who seem to need medication in order to perform in the classroom at a level consistent with their general cognitive abilities?

Here, it seems to me, we have much to discover through behavior genetics and related fields. As these fields advance in the decades ahead, we will likely discover precise ways in which human beings differ from each other, and we may learn equally precise technologies to mitigate some of these differences. If we pick up the use of these technologies without a healthy regard for the differences among human beings that underlie them, we are likely to make serious mistakes in judgment about the use of these technologies. One size pill does *not* fit all. One child may need Ritalin, but that tells us nothing about the next child's needs.

Even so, we must still ask whether it is the purpose of new technological means to mitigate the differences among human beings or to surmount handicapping conditions. Other technologies such as robotics and computers are in fact being used this way, and we expect to see even more developments in this area that already enjoys widespread approval. Will this approval extend from computers to pharmacology and genetics? Based on our experience to date with psychopharmacology, the answer appears to be yes. But even if we agreed that any new technological means may be used to surmount some aspects of handicapping conditions, we may find it very hard to know how to define a handicap or to limit the use of technology to those cases. One of the worries about Prozac is that it helps not only those who seem to need it, but those who do not.

Nevertheless, the same technology applied to different persons with different capabilities will in fact have similar but significantly different effects, and we must learn to understand as fully as possible the differences between persons and between the ways in which the same technology might affect them. Unless we as a society learn to reflect more openly than we do now on human differences and to distinguish this topic from racism and other pathologies, we might find ourselves backed into approving a technology for everyone because we want to approve it for some. As a society, we are deeply conflicted about the meaning of the differences among us. On the one hand, we affirm difference and are worried that these technologies might remove them. On the other, we seem perfectly willing to remove any differences which put people at a disadvantage. Because we are conflicted about the meaning of our differences, we are disquieted by new technological means and by the two very distinct ways in which we might use them. Should we limit some of these new means to the removal of the differences among us, and thus destroy whatever value we claim to attach to difference? Or should we ignore our differences and permit the use of these means by anyone (because, after all, we permit it for some), only to find that we have amplified our differences and piled advantage on top of advantage, making tall children taller? Then our tendency toward a "thin" description of effects would be met by our tendency to ignore differences, and the result could be a relentless technological pursuit of advantage.

## NOTES

1. For example, see W. French Anderson, "Genetic Engineering and Our Humanness," *Human Gene Therapy* 5 (1994): 755–60.

2. See Peter D. Kramer, *Listening to Prozac* (New York: Penguin Books, 1993).

3. Thomas Elbert et al., "Increased Cortical Representation of the Fingers of the Left Hand in String Players," *Science* 270 (1995):305.

4. See Thomas H. Murray, "Drugs, Sports and Ethics," in *Feeling Good and Doing Better: Ethics and Nontherapeutic Drug Use,* ed. Thomas H. Murray, Willard Gaylin, and Ruth Macklin (Clifton, New Jersey: Human Press, 1984), pp. 107–29.

MARGARET OLIVIA LITTLE

# Cosmetic Surgery, Suspect Norms, and the Ethics of Complicity

Cosmetic surgery is often cited as a paradigm of "medical enhancement."[1] Most of the time, this classification is meant to signal the view that such surgery is not medically necessary—not needed, that is, for the maintenance or restoration of health. Under one publicly popular picture of what moves people to have cosmetic surgery (what we might call the "Beverly Hills" picture), such a conclusion follows from the view that the surgery isn't necessary in any sense: it is a luxury, motivated by pleasure—and pleasure born of vanity, to boot—rather than the need to avoid or end suffering. In reality, of course, the landscape is more mixed: while there are cultural enclaves in which the pursuit of "beauty by scalpel" is as excessive as any parody might imagine, requests for cosmetic surgery are often motivated by deep and genuine suffering, in which surgery is pursued, not from a desire for beauty, but from a desire to end a distressing sense of alienation from some body part or to escape incessant teasing. In these cases, classifying cosmetic surgery as beyond medical necessity is not meant to make light of the suffering, but to remind us that the suffering is not born of disease or physiological dysfunction: whatever necessity the surgeries might carry, it is not *medical* necessity.

Questions about cosmetic surgery's status as an enhancement in this sense of the term are clearly of importance when we are trying to decide whether its provision falls within the *duties* of medical practitioners and third-party payers. But there is another set of questions about cosmetic surgery's status as an enhancement that concerns a very different, and altogether more charged, issue—namely, whether it is *appropriate* for medicine to provide it. For enhancement is also sometimes used as a boundary concept, marking off the limits of what falls within medicine's purview; and questions recur about whether cosmetic surgeries fall on the far side of that boundary. This set of questions concerns, not whether medicine must provide cosmetic surgery, but whether it *ought* to.

The question is most familiarly raised about cosmetic surgery *tout court*, expressing concern about the very idea of medicine using its interventions to alter appearances. Raised in this way, the question is familiarly controversial. Those with a traditional conception of medicine's telos will be uneasy at the thought of using surgery to satisfy the dictates of fads and fashions, of incurring medical risk without providing medical benefit. Others will argue that the source of suffering is less important than the ability of medicine to alleviate it; indeed, some will extend the argument to ask why medicine shouldn't provide a little pleasure, and not just remove pain, as long as the risks aren't too high.

While this controversy is an interesting and important one, focusing our attention on the appropriateness of cosmetic surgery as such threatens to obscure a deeper and much graver issue about medicine's involvement with the cosmetic. Whatever we think about medicine being in the general business of altering appearances, I will argue that we should have special concerns about a specific class of cosmetic surgeries— namely, those whose moral status is complicated by their relationship to what I'll be calling "suspect norms of appearance." As I will explain, this moral issue is a nuanced one that won't be resolved simply by deciding how narrowly or broadly to draw medicine's telos or by weighing the risks and benefits of procedures to individual patients. In this essay, I want to isolate the nature of the concern I have in mind, to defend that it is important, and to suggest some of the implications it carries for the contours of medicine's moral responsibilities.

## Surgery and Social Norms

Cosmetic surgery, as a class, is distinctive in that the suffering medicine is asked to alleviate is in some sense due to social attitudes and norms rather than some disease or biological dysfunction. What distinguishes the distress suffered over some aspect of one's appearance from the pain, say, of a broken leg is that the former is parasitic on some value or aesthetic norm that society happens to hold. Perhaps the patient has internalized the norm and wants very much to meet it; perhaps she herself does not accept it but suffers because those who do accept the norm treat her differently. Concerns with appearance, then, reflect the influences of social attitudes, values, and preferences. I want to urge, though, that not all norms and pressures about appearance are on the same moral plane. Let me give three sets of cases to illustrate what I have in mind.

For the first case, imagine a society in which double chins are regarded as enormously attractive. While deeply held, the preference for voluptuous chins is understood to be a matter of aesthetic taste: those who possess only one chin are not vilified; they simply aren't anyone's idea of the dream Saturday-night date. In this society, as in ours, people differ in how much importance they place on being attractive, and some will be blithely carefree about the whole issue; but we can well imagine a person who has come to suffer deeply because he has just the one lonely chin. He has tried, we shall imagine, to shrug off this lack, to find compensating measures elsewhere in his life, even psychotherapy, all to no avail. He is self-conscious and miserable with his current chin, and requests a surgical implant.

The second case is all too real. Think of a young boy who has ears that stick straight out. Imagine further that he is one of the unfortunates who is teased mercilessly and constantly by his schoolmates and children of casual encounter. His parents have tried to comfort him and to offer him strategies for dealing with his tormentors, but to no avail. The taunting has begun to color his whole outlook on life: he becomes withdrawn, begins wetting the bed; his grades drop. His parents finally decide, with his enthusiastic support and relief, to request that a surgeon tuck his ears closer to his head.

The third case is also taken from our own society. Imagine a black person who, either because he has internalized certain messages or because he wishes to escape certain stigmas, requests procedures that will make him look more like a white European—narrowing the nose, thinning the lips, lightening the skin. Or again, imagine a woman who, increasingly distressed and dissatisfied with her size-eight body and the enormous gap she perceives between that body and the pictures of feminine physicality ubiquitous in popular culture, requests a series of surgeries that will bring her closer to the paradigm exemplified by super models—extensive liposuction, recontouring the cheekbones, perhaps a rib extraction or two, all finished off with breast augmentation.

Even if we stipulate that the levels of suffering are the same in these three cases, I want to urge that they are importantly different in terms of the moral considerations they raise. Start with the first case. Hopefully we can sympathize with the poor fellow who has but one chin: given his yearning to be attractive and the aesthetic tastes of his society, we can agree that he was dealt a bad hand in life's lottery. But in this sort of case, while the person suffers real pain that is indeed importantly parasitic on his society's attitudes and preferences, I don't think we would say that society is *culpable* for that pain. Society gets to have convergences of idiosyncratic preferences, tastes, fads, and fashions. Such convergences will affect different people differently, but this difference alone does not mean that anything morally problematic is afoot. As the saying goes, not everything that is *unfortunate* is *unfair*. To give another example, in the United States more people are fanatical about basketball than about horse racing; very tall men therefore have a shot at becoming famous sports heroes in a way that very short men do not. A man whose sole desire in life is to reach mega-stardom in the sports world but who is only five feet tall has a dream that is very unlikely to come true. But again, while we may pity this person's distress and empathize with his misfortune, we should not regard it as pain that implicates society.

Turn now to the second case, to the boy whose ears stick out. Once again we find society expressing a certain preference, this time for a particular ear formation. In this case, though, something has gone wrong with society's reaction to those who deviate from the preferred appearance. Here the costs imposed for such deviation—the teasing, the ostracism—are grossly out of proportion to society's own reflective valuation of the norm. They are punitive, intolerant, in a word, *cruel*. In contrast to the first case, in which the society's aesthetic preference was strong but morally tolerant, in this case parts of society—children, say, and the parents, teachers, and other adults who are negligently permissive about the children's behavior—act immorally in the costs they mete out to those who fail to meet their preferences. We might call the attitude toward the boy a prejudice rather than a preference to mark the difference. Here society surely deserves blame for at least some of the boy's suffering—not because society has preferences or norms about appearance, but because it is immoral in its "enforcement" of those norms.

Now part of what is morally problematic about the third class of examples (illustrated by surgeries designed to make blacks look more white and women more like super models) is a similar inappropriateness in the enforcement of norms. Part of our unease about a black person being made to look more white results from the fact that the punishment inflicted on those with extremely black African features is often egregious, ranging from cruel teasing and ostracism to lessened opportunities in employment and housing. A similar story can be told for the norms of appearance that women face. While both men and women face pressures regarding their appearance, the pressures are neither symmetrical nor equal. Woman has tended historically to be *defined* by her appearance in a way man has not.[2] The virtue of beauty has been more central to female virtues than it has to male virtues, and woman has been more tightly associated or identified with body than with mind (a point that reappears historically as a premise undergirding the conclusion that woman is less rational than man).[3] Norms of appearance turn out to be, then, not norms of a *good-looking woman,* but norms of a *good woman,* full stop. Deviations from these norms of appearance are thus more highly punished than those applying to men (the pressure to "make the most of oneself" is for women a pressure that bespeaks an *obligation,* not a desideratum). After all, a man who fails in this category has failed in something that is only incidental to his nature; a woman has sinned against one of her deepest charges.

Part of what is morally problematic about the third class of cases, then, is that the cost imposed by society for failing to live up to its norms of appearance is here excessive, punitive, unfair, or cruel. But this problem isn't, I think, the full story about the third class of cases. I want to argue that there is another, very important source of moral unease in this third category. What is also problematic about these surgeries, I want to urge, is that the very *content* of the norms of appearance they involve is morally suspect. We feel a heightened moral unease about these cases, I want to urge, because the norms of appearance at issue are grounded in or get life from a broader system of attitudes and actions that is in fact *unjust.*

Consider the norm of attractiveness at issue in surgeries designed to make blacks look more white. We are not dealing here with some whimsical aesthetic preference. It is no *accident* that the standard of beauty prevalent in the West favors white European features over black African ones. It reflects a long-standing tradition in which being black is devalued and being white is valorized. Indeed, it reflects the remnants of a time-honored view—supported through history by major social institutions, especially science and religion—that the races are hierarchically arranged in nature, with the white race standing as the exemplar of humanity, while the black race, quite literally subhuman, stands closer to the apes.[4] The racial and ethnic contours of our norms of attractiveness were shaped as part and parcel of this broader conception of humanity.

Our uneasiness at the example of the black trying to look more white, then, is not simply a result of the fact that it involves racial features. There is something more presumptively problematic about incentives and pressures for blacks to look white than there is about incentives and pressures for whites to play with the exoticism of looking black. The former takes place against a broad context of devaluing blackness and a pressure to assimilate to an unjust paradigm of humanness.

Once again the point continues with the norms of appearance that are applied to women. Throughout history, woman and the "feminine" has been cast in roles of contamination, infection, and danger.[5] The resulting alienation toward features regarded as distinctly or especially feminine gets reflected in the norms of appearance applying to the feminine: in some cultures, it appears as a hatred of female fat, in others, as a hatred of female body hair. In virtually all cultures, it shows up in the fact that women's norms of appearance tend to be farther from the natural, the average, or the usual than are men's (e.g. fewer decades of a woman's life than a man's count as candidates for beauty)— a point that helps explain why women's standards of appearance are usually much harder to meet than are men's. Further, as several historians have noted, the idea of beauty has been defined as the object of the male, not female, gaze.[6] Given that the nature and worth of woman are seen as residing so largely in her appearance, subliminally we begin to believe that the nature and worth of woman reside largely, if not exhaustively, in her existence as an object of male gaze. Consequently, the content of women's norms of appearance have a much greater tendency to objectify women than do men's norms of appearance—a theoretical point that is borne out all too vividly when we look at images of women in "entertainment" and advertising.[7] At heart, the norms of women's appearance reflect, not aesthetic whim, but distorted, unjust conceptions of woman herself.

In the third classification, then, the content of the standards is part and parcel of an unjust social ideology. The examples so far adduced have involved race and gender, but I don't mean to suggest that the problem is limited to these categories. Put generally, it seems to me that norms of appearance occupy a morally suspect status when their content reflects, flows from, and reinforces a system of beliefs, attitudes, and practices that together involve deep injustice. If any one central theme is common to such oppressive systems, as we might call them, it is perhaps the view that some group occupies less than full human status; and certainly categories other than race and gender have been the target of such ideological exclusions. Take for instance the case of children with Down's syndrome. Such children have distinctive facial features that publicly "mark" them; as such they often encounter hurtful teasing and distorted expectations. At the very least such cases belong in our second category, as instances in which society is culpably cruel in the costs it imposes for failing to meet some norm. But such cases may also fit the third category, for the *content* of the norms invoked may well be morally suspect. That is, while it may be that we have a merely aesthetic dislike of the facial features typical of those with Down's syndrome, it may be that the reason we have such an aesthetic reaction is because of some historical association these features have with a certain conception of "idiocy," namely, one in which "idiots" were regarded as occupying something less than full human status. The extent to which such a conception continues subterraneously to inform those norms, and for the norms to reinforce a broader system of unfairly constraining practices, is the extent to which the content of the norms themselves inherit a status that is morally suspect.

The cases of cosmetic surgery that raise special moral concern, then, are cases in which the dissatisfaction or distress that people ask medicine to alleviate results, not from morally innocuous preferences, but from practices or ideologies that are morally troubling—for instance, suffering that stems from cruel teasing, or distress that arises from trying to meet the pressures of a norm whose content is steeped in injustice. The question now at issue is whether this concern is one that is relevant to the moral responsibilities of *medicine*. Does the fact that the demand for such surgeries arises in problematic contexts count as a morally salient consideration for medicine's practices; does it carry any ethical implications for medicine as an institution or for surgeons as individual professionals?

One mainstream view of medicine's responsibilities contends that it does not. According to this view, much as we may abhor the attitudes and pressures that lie behind such surgeries, it is not and cannot be within medicine's purview to pass judgment on them or to use them as factors in determining what surgeries should be performed. After all, it is urged, to perform a surgery is not to agree with the values underwriting the request—physicians often disagree with patients' values or preferences, but respect for patient autonomy requires that they not automatically substitute their own values for the patient's. In short, while the moral unease we feel at surgeries designed to make blacks look more white or women look more like super models may point to an important agenda for general society, medicine's role-specific duty must be to bracket these concerns, to take the situation as it is found, and to focus on its primary charge: having compassion for patients' suffering and alleviating it where possible.

However appealing such a view is on first glance, it fails to do justice to the moral contours of the situation. Whatever we might decide about the all-things-considered moral permissibility of performing such surgeries, we must surely agree that they call for *some* sort of moral hesitancy. That is, a surgeon who finds herself in a community of Stepford women trying to look pneumatic, or in a racist state whose government pays for blacks to look more white, must surely feel some moral unease at using her role to such purposes. To put it somewhat differently, even if the surgeon decides to go ahead with the surgeries— to alleviate, say, the extreme censure the patients would otherwise face—there will be a moral *residue* to doing so. But the model of medical responsibility that underwrites this response provides no means for explaining or grounding this modest, and thoroughly intuitive, notion. Even if the suspect nature of the norms leaves the surgeries permissible, it is far too strong to say that it is of no moral salience to the surgeon at all.

I think that the mainstream model gets the wrong answer because it's looking in the wrong place. It assumes that the moral covenant at issue in these worrisome surgeries is the surgeon's covenant to the individual patients who stand before her. It casts the moral question, that is, in terms of the physician-patient relationship, an approach which, not surprisingly, delivers the familiar advice to alleviate the patient's suffering and respect his autonomy wherever possible. But the moral complication such surgeries present to medicine concerns another relationship altogether—the relation between the surgeon, or indeed medicine as an institution, and the suspect norms and practices themselves. We focus the moral issue too tightly if we focus only on the duty to relieve suffering, for as real as this duty is, there is a further issue about the physician's relationship to the system that causes that suffering. The deeper moral issue these cosmetic surgeries raise is, in short, the issue of *complicity*.

## Acting with Integrity

What is it permissible to do in the face of cruel bullying or of pressures backed by suspect norms? When is it acceptable to accommodate these pressures, and when does doing so count as "selling out" or "giving in"? What paths from suffering can one take without a loss of integrity? When is one to be cheered for taking measures to escape the unfairly punitive system, and when is one to be judged an "Uncle Tom" or a "recruit of the patriarchy"? These questions hopefully give some indication of the complexity of the moral terrain here. Concerns about complicity are *nuanced* concerns. They are not reducible to moral concerns about the aggregate net utility of one's actions, or to concerns about the wrongs one might do to some specified individuals. To be complicitous is to bear some improper relation *to the evil* of some practice or set of attitudes. Just what relation is it?

Put in broadest brushstrokes, let me suggest that one is complicitous when one endorses, promotes, or unduly benefits from norms and practices that are morally suspect. How we unpack this schematic answer depends on the context, of course. Certainly, the worst cases are those that involve explicit (if sometimes subtle) endorsement and exploitation of the norms and practices themselves. In the practice of cosmetic surgery, we find this sort of crass complicity represented all too well. The widespread practices of advertising to create demand, of underemphasizing risks and overclaiming results, of suggesting procedures over and above the ones initially requested by the patient, are bad enough; the point here is that the promotions often exploit the suspect norms themselves. When the surgeries suggested to blacks are predictably for narrower noses rather than broader ones, when advertisement rhetoric plays to women's anxieties that anything over size four is fat, when patients report that surgeons suggest breast augmentations more often than they suggest breast reduction, we have patterns that reflect and endorse the content of the suspect norms. Matters are worse when such exploitation is done for the purpose of personal gain. Whether or not medicine in general should be pursued simply to make money (an issue I'm bracketing here), performing surgeries involving suspect norms solely for personal gain deserves heightened scrutiny—think of acting the Uncle Tom to make one's *second* million. Indeed, whatever the motive, there is something presumptively troubling about a practice that reaps profit from making society more white and women more like Barbie Dolls, if only because those who profit from the system run a tremendous danger of becoming invested in seeing it continue.

There are, then, cases in which practitioners of medicine have, in essence, "sided" with the suspect norms of appearance, exploiting their content and counterfactually sustaining their force. These cases deserve our ethical scrutiny and our ethical censure. But the theoretically more challenging, because more subtle, aspect of complicity remains yet to be addressed. Obviously, the picture presented here, while depressingly common, does not describe all cosmetic surgeons. Just as patients have a variety of motives for requesting cosmetic surgery, not all of which fit stereotypes of shallow vanity, surgeons have a variety of motives for performing such surgeries, not all of which fit stereotypes of cynical exploitation. Many surgeons are morally decent folk—a few even morally heroic—whose intentions betray no endorsement of the norms that underwrite many patients' requests. They decry the pressures that lead to patients' suffering, much as they would decry the prevalence of a virus, and would change that aspect of society if they could; in the meantime, though, they are motivated by the genuinely noble goal of relieving the distress they find. (Indeed, the now-classic moral defense for performing frivolous or worrisome cosmetic surgeries is that it funds *pro bono* work doing reconstructive surgery on those with severe disfigurements.)

Certainly, we want to mark off these activities as different from the crass ones. But the deeper question is whether the difference is sufficient to free them from all dangers of complicity. The question is whether purity of motive suffices to insulate actions. Take, for instance, first-person worries about one's own possible complicity. Such questions only arise when one abhors a system—one wouldn't *worry* about participating in an activity one endorsed. The surgeon who is asked to make blacks look more like whites under a system of apartheid feels tension at the prospect of performing such surgeries precisely *because* she regards apartheid as evil. Questions about complicity often start, not end, with the judgment that one disapproves of a system or practice. Reflecting on these points presses us to question whether an approach that grants us absolution from complicity as long as we don't want to support a suspect system might be drawing the moral lines too cleanly.

The residual concern is that complicity might arise, not just when one subjectively endorses the suspect system, but when one's actions in fact end up reinforcing it. Clearly, one's actions can de facto serve to promote a system one does not intentionally set out to bolster, and the danger is particularly deep for the actions of medicine. For one thing, medicine enjoys an extraordinarily high institutional status in society; its participation in such surgeries can easily be regarded as sanctioning the importance and appropriateness of those norms. When the institution of medicine helps turn society white or women into

Barbie Dolls, those maneuvers can seem to be backed by one of the central institutional authorities of our society. Further danger arises from the fact that the institution of medicine, in addition to occupying high status, is primarily concerned with health and healing. Its participation can unwittingly bring suspect surgeries under that umbrella, so that the norms of appearance get blurred with norms of "health" and "normalcy," reinforcing sexist and racist conceptions of what the paradigm human is like. And the mere fact that medical interventions, which in general are associated with risk and invasiveness, are used to achieve some end tends to elevate the importance of that end: the tacit inference is that it must be *worth* doing, and not simply idiosyncratically desired, if it justifies taking such risks. (This outcome is especially true when surgeries are designed merely to gratify a patient's desire to meet the norm. When the deployment of medicine's social role is not the alleviation of suffering, but the satisfaction of the desire to meet a norm of appearance, the norm itself becomes elevated in stature—the opposite of what we want to see happen when the norms are suspect.)

But what are the contours of moral responsibility here? Are we now to conclude that duty demands us to avoid anything that will causally reinforce a suspect system? Do our own conceptions of our actions count for nothing? If we are tempted by the view that intention is the sole arbiter of complicity, it is surely in part because we recoil at the thought that the morality of our actions should be held hostage in this way to the existence of the suspect system, which would end up not only causing harm but grounding a startling extensive prohibition against measures that might help alleviate that harm.

The question here is what counts as "participating in" a suspect system one does not endorse; and it misses the nuance of complicity simply to equate that notion with causal reinforcement of a system. For the nuance of complicity (and the reason I think it is such a useful concept) is located precisely in the fact that responsibility for such causal effect should sometimes be laid at our doorstep and sometimes at the doorstep of the suspect system.

Let me suggest a different approach to the issue. When even well-intentioned actions unwittingly play a large role in legitimizing and reinforcing the suspect norms under discussion, they do so because of the *meaning* that those surgeries carry for others—they do so because others see in them a legitimization of or pressure to meet norms. This approach gives us better direction for understanding the terrain of responsibilities here. Clearly, one should not be held hostage to all possible interpretations of our actions, to all the meanings others might attach to our behavior. But it is negligence to ignore the interpretations that others may naturally be expected to place on our actions given the broad context in which they take place. That is, while one is not responsible, for instance, when others willfully or negligently misinterpret one's actions, one cannot simply turn a blind eye to all but the meanings one *wishes* others would see in our actions: we have a duty to forestall those interpretations that, while unintended, would be completely natural given the larger background context in which the action takes place.

If something like this notion is right, then the key to analyzing complicity is found when we remember that the meaning carried by actions, just as the meaning carried by words, is determined *holistically*. It is not found in individual features of an action—it is not equivalent to its effects, and it is certainly not solipsistically determined by our intention. Meaning emerges, rather, as a function of a broad context, including, significantly, the backdrop of other actions one performs. This idea suggests that we refocus our moral attention. Instead of examining the morality of an individual piece of surgery, we must examine the context in which that individual act of surgery takes place. The broad implication is, in essence, a conditional form of the motto, "If you're not part of the solution, you're part of the problem." If one must perform surgeries to help people meet suspect norms of appearance (out of concern for their suffering, say), then one must maintain an overall stance of fighting the norms. The only way to participate in the surgeries without de facto promoting the evil whose effects one decries is to locate the surgery in a broader context of naming and rejecting the evil norms. One's purpose and meaning—that of alleviating the extreme burdens the system places on some—can be expressed only if one's broader actions stand squarely against the norms.

Even in pursuing surgery from motives that are distant from the suspect norms, then, one must be cognizant of, and take into account, the possible side effects of one's actions. One has a responsibility to maintain and make clear the meaning of the action, and to factor in the increased pressure others may in fact feel as a result of having surgically "improved" appearance. At the very least, this responsibility would require those who perform the surgeries to speak out publicly against the suspect content of the norms—to be a general voice against, rather than promoter of, the norms and practices in question. But it will also issue in more specific recommendations driven by the specific contours of the suspect system's content. Let me give an example drawing from the case of women's appearance.

A true appreciation of the special injustices underlying norms of women's appearance would influence and enrichen our idea of what constitutes proper informed consent for such surgeries. Take for instance the matter of informing patients of the options they face. It may seem needless to recount the option of not pursuing surgery, but in fact doing so is not at all unimportant. One of the insidious ways sexism works is by gradually constricting the options that women imaginatively conceive for themselves. Such constriction happens, of course, with women's norms of appearance: the presumption for certain appearances is so heavy that our models of acceptable appearance occupy a narrow range. Medicine can take proactive steps to counteract this constriction by responsibly underscoring the option not to pursue surgery.

I don't mean that medicine should issue some vague admonition for women to rest content with their current appearance: to do so would be naive if not condescending. But far more use could be made of women's own differing experiences with cosmetic surgery and appearance. Some prospective patients arrive at medicine's doorstep less decided on the procedures than others. It would help stretch their imaginative options if one gave these women access (through videos, conversations, or written narratives) to a wide variety of women's experience: experiences from women who decided to go through with the surgery and are happy, from those who did so and have regrets, and from women who decided in the end not to have the surgery at all. And, again, it is important for women to have access to studies and narratives that bring to life the various real-life experiences women have of their bodies and society's reaction to them, not only that benefits are portrayed more realistically, but that the dangers and risks—social as well as medical—are understood. To give just one example, some defend breast augmentation as empowering, for large breasts enable one to "rivet men's gaze."[8] But it is not the power to rivet men's gaze when and only when one desires that gaze, and there are many circumstances in which having a man's gaze riveted at one's breasts is anything but what one desires, as when one is trying to be taken seriously as a job candidate.

## *Conclusion*

Whatever we think of the general idea of medicine altering appearance, we should have special, and deep, concerns about medicine participating in practices that reflect and reinforce certain suspect norms of appearance. Medicine and surgeons must beware the extent to which their participation in cosmetic surgeries involving such norms ends up contributing to a broad and unjust system of constraining pressures and forces. For while we want to alleviate what can be very real pain, the danger arises that, in doing so, we will be acting in a way that is complicitous with the very evils that give rise to it.

Yet there is surely some role for medicine to perform surgeries even in cases involving suspect norms. There is a limit to the suffering we require victims of the norm to bear before taking measures to escape that suffering, and health care professionals are sometimes the only ones who can alleviate that distress. Determining medicine's proper role in helping people meet suspect norms of appearance, then, is a complicated task, for there are two relations a physician must properly juggle—her relation to the individual patient, and her relation to the system of norms.

The tension between the duties grounded in these respective relations, I have argued, can be somewhat lessened when we remember that the relation one must maintain to the norms is *holistically* defined: one must, if one participates in such surgeries at all, maintain an overall stance of fighting against the system. Such a general stance can leave room for occasions of helping a distressed patient by performing surgery that admittedly involves the suspect norms. There is all the difference in the world, that is, between, on the one hand, a surgeon who promotes, suggests, and aggressively advertises these surgeries, who performs them whether the patient requests it out of self-abnegation, desire for power, or anguish, who is glad when, for instance, trends in women's figures and faces change because shifting fads mean repeat business, and who is vaguely pleased that there is so much pressure on women to meet the norms because it means increased profits, and, on the other hand, a surgeon who does not suggest or promote the suspect surgeries, who helps her patients explore other options, who speaks out against the pressures women face, but who occasionally uses her surgical skills in cases where there seems no other path out of true suffering. Medicine does indeed have two duties to attend to when thinking about whether to perform the troubling surgeries, but I think they can be somewhat reconciled: sometimes perform the surgery, and always fight the system.

## NOTES

1. This article is a companion piece to my article, "Suspect Norms of Appearance and the Ethics of Complicity," in *In the Eye of the Beholder: Ethics and Medical Change of Appearance*, ed. Inez de Beaufort, Medard Hilhorst, and Soren Holm (Scandinavian University Press, 1997), pp. 151–67; some paragraphs in this essay are taken from that article.

2. See Sandra Lee Bartky, *Femininity and Domination: Studies in the Phenomenology of Oppression* (New York and London: Routledge, 1990), especially chapters 3 and 5; Susan Bordo, *Unbearable Weight: Feminism, Western Culture, and the Body* (Berkeley: University of California Press, 1993).

3. Sherry Ortner, "Is Female to Nature as Male Is to Culture?" in *Women, Culture and Society,* ed. Michelle Zimbalist and Louise Lamphere (Stanford: Stanford University Press, 1974); Carolyn Merchant, *The Death of Nature* (San Francisco: Harper and Row, 1980); Genevieve Lloyd, "Reason, Gender, and Morality in the History of Philosophy," *Social Research* 50, no. 3 (Autumn 1983): 490–513.

4. For examples and discussion, see Stephen Jay Gould, *The Mismeasure of Man* (New York and London: W.W. Norton & Co., 1981).

5. See Merchant, *The Death of Nature*, and Lloyd, "Reason, Gender, and Morality."

6. Arthur Marwick, *Beauty in History* (London: Thames and Hudson, 1988); Reena N. Glazer, "Women's Body Image and the Law," *Duke Law Journal* 43 (1993): 113–47.

7. See Susan Bordo, *Unbearable Weight*.

8. I am indebted to my colleague Alisa Carse for the example and skeptical analysis.

CARL ELLIOTT

# The Tyranny of Happiness: Ethics and Cosmetic Psychopharmacology

"Cosmetic psychopharmacology" is a term of art invented by Peter Kramer in his book *Listening to Prozac*. Prozac, of course, is an antidepressant, but what is so intriguing about it is not what it does for patients who are clinically depressed but what it does for those who aren't: patients who are shy and withdrawn, or who are rather compulsive, or who have poor self-esteem, or who are just plain chronically sad. What Kramer found was that when he put some of these patients on Prozac (but not all or even most of them), they underwent a kind of personality transformation. The controlling, compulsive types became laid-back and easygoing; shy people became more self-confident and assertive. Lonely hearts went on Prozac and pretty soon they had three dates a weekend. It is this kind of effect that Kramer calls cosmetic psychopharmacology, and it worries him. And what worries him is not something as simple as Prozac making sad people happier but less interesting or less creative. What is more deeply worrying is that for at least some of the patients on Prozac, their personality changes really do seem to be for the better. Kramer's patients say things like, "I feel like I've been drugged all my life and now I'm finally clear-headed," or, "I never really felt like myself until now." Some patients seem to be able to see themselves in a way that they had been incapable of before. They don't just get well; they say, "I'm better than well."

There are lots of questions to be answered here, empirical questions about how often these personality transformations actually happen, and philosophical questions about the difference between curing a mental illness and enhancing your personality. But what interests me is another question, which is rather different. Some of the patients that both Kramer and other psychiatrists describe are a special sort. These are people who are empty and confused, sad or lonely people whose lives don't seem to have any direction, people like Kramer's patients who say things like "I don't know who I am," or "The whole world seems to be in on something that I just don't get."[1] These people sound strikingly like the alienated Southern heroes in Walker Percy's novels, like Will Barrett in *The Last Gentleman*, a prosperous young Southerner who looks at all the prosperous Southerners around him and says, "Why do I feel so bad when they all feel so good? Why do I feel better holding a shotgun than a three-iron?" Percy's most direct statement on this question comes, of course, in his satire *Love in the Ruins*, whose psychiatrist-hero Tom More invents what he calls a stethoscope of the human soul, the Ontological Lapsometer, which can diagnose and treat these existential illnesses. So I want to concentrate on just this one particular sort of worry about cosmetic Prozac, the worry that Percy had, which comes down to something like this: suppose we could relieve all these patients of their sense of spiritual emptiness or alienation, these people who feel disoriented and lost in the world. Would that be a good thing, or is it sometimes better to feel bad than to feel good?

Now when some people try to articulate why it might sometimes be better to feel bad than to feel good, they often say that anxiety or depression is part of the human condition, or part of what it means to be human. That may be right, but it is not what I want to say. What I want to say is not about human beings in general but about human beings in the West in the twentieth century, and the predicament that many of us find ourselves in.

All human beings, no matter where or when they live, live within certain frameworks of understanding that give sense to their actions and to their lives. As Charles Taylor points out, they include understandings about what sort of lives have dignity, what counts as a good life and what counts a failure, what kind of life is worth living, and most important for us, when a life has meaning, or sense. We could call these frameworks transcendent in that they involve a kind of orientation toward a higher good or goods that are independent of our own will, or preferences, desires. Taylor, for example, develops a concept that he calls "strong evaluation."[2] Strong evaluation is not about what we happen to prefer or have an interest in, but about what we think that people would be the worse for not preferring or having an interest in. So I would not think worse of a person if, say, he thought Dickens was a better writer than Tolstoy, even though I might think that he was wrong. But I might well think worse of him if he thinks that novels are a waste of time. I once heard Pauline Kael say on the radio that she couldn't really be friends with anyone who liked the movie "Forrest Gump." That's a strong evaluation, but it is also a kind of trivial aesthetic evaluation. What I have in mind are the kind of serious *ethical* evaluations that we make when we say, for instance, that a person is wasting his life.

How does this notion relate to our predicament as 20th century Westerners? In other times and other cultures a person might worry about his life being a failure *within* a given framework of understanding— about failing to meet the demands of his station in life, or of losing his honor, or of failing to live a life that will get him admitted into heaven, or displeasing his ancestors, and so on. Very often we feel some of these demands ourselves. But modern, twentieth-century Westerners face another problem: not that of failing to meet the demands of one's framework, like a Southern gentleman who backs down from a duel, but of being unsure of what the framework is. This uncertainty is an altogether new and frightening kind of feeling, a feeling Taylor compares to vertigo: a sense of imbalance, because not only don't you know what kind of life to live; you don't know what, if anything, can tell you.

Now people experience this feeling in different ways: as vertigo, absurdity, emptiness, the malaise. And when we try to articulate it we ask questions like: Is this all there is? What is the sense of life? How does it all fit together? But Walker Percy puts his finger on the way the question appears to many of us, which is What am I supposed to be doing? This is not idle philosophizing: it is a practical question about action. Who am I supposed to be, and what am I supposed to do next? Percy's characters are more often than not Southerners who don't really fit in the South. Sometimes they get a kind of nostalgia, or false nostalgia, for the old antebellum South, the stoic South where their grandfathers lived, not because they ever knew those times or even think they were especially enlightened but because at least then honor was honor and sin was sin and a person knew where he stood.

Let me try to make an analogy between this deep sense of existential imbalance that Percy writes about and a similar but shallower variant that may be more common. I was born and raised in the South, but over the past nine years I have lived in five different countries. Each time I come back to the South after a period away I feel slightly disoriented. Things are pretty much the same, but they *feel* different, even slightly foreign. Little things, of course, like having children say "yes sir" when they address me, and being expected to go to church on Sunday, but also the larger patterns in which people live their lives. I feel a little like an anthropologist in my own country. What I once took for granted as the way to live now seems arbitrary, just one form of life among many, and perhaps not even the best one. And this seems to cut its legs out from under it. Something like this, I suspect, is going on with this deeper, more radical sense of alienation. It is not just questioning the givenness of one's own form of life; it is questioning whether *any* form of life can have the kind of justification that you feel you need. It is a sense that all our ethical and epistemological practices are up for grabs.

So my question is this: suppose you are a psychiatrist and you have a patient who has precisely this sense of alienation; say, an accountant living in Downers Grove, Illinois who comes to himself one day and says, Jesus Christ, is this it? A Snapper lawn mower and a house in the suburbs? Should you, his psychiatrist, try to rid him of his alienation by prescribing Prozac? Or do you secretly think that maybe, as bad off as he is, he is better off than his neighbors? Because, as Percy puts it, even though he's in a predicament, at least he's aware of it, which is a lot better than being in a predicament and thinking you're not.

Now obviously, how you answer this question is going to turn on how you see the culture around him. Some societies seem to call for a response of alienation. I felt a little like this when I lived in South Africa, for example. If you see American society as hopelessly shallow, or materialistic, or unjust, then you are going to say that if a person doesn't feel radically alienated and dissatisfied and out of step, then something really *is* wrong with him.

Your response about treatment is also going to depend on whether you see this ailment as a medical problem. Some people are tempted to say: if Prozac fixes it, the problem must be biological. In fact, Kramer suggests in the last chapter of his book that Percy would have realized the value of cosmetic Prozac, perhaps even endorsed it, if he had just realized that what he thought were spiritual problems were, in fact, biological problems. I don't think so. What Percy was trying to do was to show that to treat existential problems, like alienation, as scientific problems is a kind of category mistake. In other words, if a person is depressed by the emptiness of life as an American consumer, you are missing the point completely if you try to see this as a psychiatric issue. Seeing this as a psychiatric issue is like seeing holy communion as a dietary issue. It is not completely off-base, but at bottom you have misunderstood what is really going on.

But what is going on? What, in fact, does it mean to say this is an existential problem, not a psychiatric problem? The point I am moving toward is that some of these worries that Percy had about the Ontological Lapsometer, and which some of us seem to have about cosmetic Prozac, have their roots in our own particular form of life, and in particular, about that framework within which we think of our lives as having sense or meaning. For lack of a better term, I will follow writers like Taylor and Lionel Trilling and call this framework an ethic of authenticity.[3]

I want to point out just a few features of this ethic that I think are widely held in our culture. The first is what we might call, following Michael Walzer, the notion of life as a project.[4] By the notion of life as a project I mean two related things. First is the idea that whether our lives make sense or have significance is largely up to us; that the sense or significance of our lives depends on how we live them. This idea, that how we live our lives will determine their significance, is in turn tied to a second idea: that our lives are planned undertakings which, to a large extent, we control and for which we are responsible. External factors play a part in our lives, most of us will acknowledge— luck, fate, karma, deity—but not so much that we feel ourselves exonerated from overall responsibility for the shape that our lives take.

Now we tend to take for granted this picture of our lives as our projects, but in fact it is not at all a universal picture. Think, for example, of the idea of life as something that is entrusted to you and determined by God, so that the purpose of your life is to follow God's will. The result is not a picture of life as something that we control and are responsible for, but a picture of life as something that is *given* to us; not something that we create, but something that is given, whose contours we fill in. Or take, for example, the idea that you inherit your life from your parents, and your purpose is to take over their position and social station and accomplishments. This idea does not fit a picture of your life as essentially *your* project, as we tend to think here in America, but a life lived in historical time for your parents and for your children; not life as an individual project, but as a collective project taking place over generations. When advertisers use slogans such as, "You only go around once in life," they are playing on this cultural sense we Americans tend to share: first, of our lives as disconnected from a larger historical context, and second, that our lives are essentially what we make of them.

The second feature of this contemporary ethic I want to point out concerns the content of the good life. An ethic of authenticity says that in order to answer the question, "How should I live?" I will have to look inward, because there is no single universal way of living a meaningful life. The answer to this question will differ from one person to the next, and each person has to discover the answer for himself. "You have to find yourself," we sometimes hear. "You have to find your own way." "You have to be true to yourself." Each "self" is different and unique; for a life to be a good life, a meaningful life, a life properly oriented toward the good, we have to get in touch with ourselves.

How does this ethic of authenticity relate to Prozac and the worries that we might have about it? First, if the meaningful life is connected to the authentic life, the life that is uniquely yours, then the possibility arises to live an inauthentic life. Many people would think that an inauthentic life is somehow a wasted life, or a life that failed to meet its potential—a Gauguin who didn't go to Tahiti, or perhaps closer to the mark, the life of someone who is play-acting at something he isn't, like a German who idealizes the life of the American Indians and consequently spends his weekends in the Bavarian countryside wearing a loin cloth and living in a teepee. Not that there is anything wrong about this kind of life, of course; the problem comes only if it is not truly *your* life. An unease with this kind of inauthenticity lies at the root of some of the worries that some people have about Prozac. It would be worrying if Prozac altered my personality, even if it gave me a better personality, simply because it isn't *my* personality. This kind of personality change seems to defy an ethic of authenticity.

Yet the very idea of an authentic self is slippery. Can we really say that Prozac has moved a person away from her authentic self, or her true personality, if, like Kramer's patients, she says she feels like herself only when she is on the drug? If a patient says "I don't feel like myself anymore" when she discontinues the drug, it is tempting to argue, as Kramer does, that Prozac doesn't simply change the self so much as restore the true self, the self that has been masked or hidden by pathology. However one chooses to construct these changes, either as a derangement or as a restoration of a true self, the vocabulary with which the changes are discussed (by Kramer as well as by many people who have taken Prozac) bears testimony to how deeply the notion of a true or authentic self is embedded in our culture.

Second, this ethic of authenticity connects the meaningful life in a crucial way to the individual. What becomes very important is the uniqueness of a life. Many Americans start to feel a greater sense of meaninglessness as they come to feel their lives are not unique. The natural home for the American novel of alienation is the generic, faceless suburb. I think this, for Walker Percy, was very important, and lay behind some of his own reservations about psychiatry as a whole, and why he had more confidence, in fact, in the novel as a way of dealing with alienation. Percy's insight was that if you are alienated and empty and lost in the world, then you will very likely find it therapeutic, in a very peculiar and backhanded way, to read a novel about a person who is alienated and empty and lost in the world. As Percy put it in his famous essay, there is a difference between a commuter on a train who feels bad without knowing why and that very same commuter reading a book about a man who feels bad without knowing why.[5] Whereas, as Percy didn't add but might have, there is no difference between the commuter who feels bad without knowing why and the same commuter reading a copy of DSM-IV.

Part of the reason for this difference is simply that a novel validates the reader's predicament. By describing your predicament, the novelist certifies it as something legitimate and real. Now DSM-IV does this, too, of course, by giving your illness a name, but there is a radical difference between the way the novelist looks at the man who feels bad and doesn't know why and the way that medicine ordinarily does. Binx Bolling is going to look very different in the pages of *The Moviegoer* than he would in the *Archives of General Psychiatry*. That difference is this: the medical standpoint looks at the man who feels bad and doesn't know why and says: this fellow is in a fix. He's in bad shape. What he needs is to get in therapy, develop his self-esteem, get a prescription for Prozac. Whereas what the novel says, more often than not, is sure, this guy is in bad shape; but doesn't it look better than the alternative? The novel and the movie celebrate the man's predicament, in a perverse way. Sure, Tom More is a depressed lust-ridden mental patient who drinks vodka with his grits, but who would you rather be: him, or his Presbyterian wife? The novel says, of course you're depressed. Take a look around you; it would take a moron not to be depressed.

The novel can also do things that a scientific approach to alienation can't do. This relates to the reason why Percy would say that this is an existential problem rather than a psychiatric problem. Any scientific approach to alienation is going to say something about alienation in general—about the characteristics that most alienated people share. The aim of the novelist, however, unless he is a very bad novelist, is to say something not about alienation in general but about a particular person in a particular circumstance. Not Anyone Anywhere, but Binx Bolling, a moviegoer living in Gentilly—whose subjective experience we have access to through the novel. This is a very neat trick. Percy realizes that if you're alienated, it is often precisely because you feel as if you are Anyone Anywhere, an exemplar of the type: Alienated American. And if you are Anyone Anywhere, it is not going to help your condition a bit to hear yourself described as a specimen of a type that lacks inclusivity and meaningful relationships and has not actualized his creative potential. Whereas if a novelist tells you not about the Alienated American type but about Binx Bolling, a stockbroker living in Gentilly, who, now that you mention it, seems to be in very much the same predicament as you, well, then you may start to feel a little less bad.

Which brings me to my last point, and that is the connection between an ethic of authenticity and the idea of self-fulfillment. Self-fulfillment is an essential constituent of a meaningful life. To many Americans that might sound like a commonplace, but in fact it is very different from an ethic that says your life is meaningful if you have done your duty, or pleased God, or met the demands of honor. And of course, nowadays we think that self-fulfillment involves discovering and pursuing your own values and your own particular talents—for example, though a career. I should point out that in this sense a career isn't simply a matter of selfishness, or narcissism, or even of being free to do your own thing; it's a kind of moral ideal. And what makes it a moral ideal, as Taylor points out, is not just that many people sacrifice their relationships or the care of their children or other important things for the sake of their careers. People have always done that. What is different is that now they feel *called* to do this. They feel as if they would be wasting their lives if they didn't. They feel that this kind of life is a *higher* life.

This notion is related, of course, to the idea that interests Max Weber so much in *The Protestant Ethic and the Spirit of Capitalism*. What interests Weber is not just that people will work harder to get more money, but that work takes on this moral character. Weber traced this idea to Luther's conception of a calling, where the way to please God was not to renounce the world for the monastery, but to immerse yourself in worldly affairs and fulfill the duties that the world imposes on you. This immersion was your calling. The exemplar of this attitude toward work as a moral ideal was, for Weber, the United States, with Benjamin Franklin as a kind of patron saint. What Weber saw in Franklin's writings was that wasting time or losing money was not treated as simply foolishness, or bad business, but as an ethical lapse, as a kind of moral failing. Even now I think that this idea is something that particularly strikes a lot of Europeans who visit the States; it is not that Americans necessarily work harder (Germans work hard, too), but that Americans seem to feel guilty or ashamed if they are not working. So much so, in fact, that they feel driven to pretend that they are extremely busy even if they are not.

Now I think this work ethic has played itself out in America in interesting ways. We Americans still place a high value on work in, for example, Taylor's "strongly evaluative" sense, and see the life of work as a duty, but not as duty to God; rather, as a duty to ourselves. What Luther referred to as a calling survives nowadays not so much as a calling by God, but as a calling from *within*: the idea of discovering yourself, of finding your own particular place in the world. A meaningful life is a personally fulfilling life, and fulfillment is something that you discover and create on your own, especially through the life of work, and the life of family and household.

Many contemporary Americans find the ties between work, self-fulfillment, and the meaningful life self-evident. As T.J. Jackson Lears has pointed out in his dazzling study of American antimodernism, these ties have deep roots in American culture.[6] Lears sees the ties between work and the meaningful life not merely in such familiar American images as the industrious, disciplined, "self-made man" of nineteenth-century success mythology—a man motivated as much by ethics and ideology as by material reward—but also in less obvious intellectual currents, such as the Arts and Crafts movement that flourished around the turn of the century. Recoiling from the factories and bureaucracies of organized capitalism, craft idealogues extolled the nobility, even the holiness, of honest, creative work. That work had a deeply spiritual character was obvious to craft revivalists such as Horace Traubel, co-founder of the Pennsylvania agrarian community Rose Valley, which offered a return to a simpler, more "authentic" way of life. At Rose Valley, as Traubel tellingly put it, "work was worship, the workbench an altar, and bad work blasphemy."[7]

We can see something of these ideas in the conflicted attitudes that many Americans have toward Prozac. On the one hand, if the way to lead a meaningful life is to search for self-fulfillment, and self-fulfillment is achieved through a life of honest work and householding, then it makes sense to embrace a drug like Prozac, which offers the promise of doing better, more meaningful work in a happier, more enthusiastic way. Yet if living a meaningful life is also tied to living an authentic life—the life that is uniquely yours, which you discover and develop by looking inward—then a drug like Prozac can seem deeply problematic. What could seem less authentic, at least on the surface, than changing your personality with an antidepressant? What could be further from the "simple life" than a life dependent on cosmetic psychopharmacology?

In some ways, the relationship of cosmetic Prozac to an ethic of authenticity is similar to that of psychedelic drugs like mescaline and LSD in the 1950s and 1960s.[8] For intellectuals like Aldous Huxley, psychedelic drugs were a powerful tool in the search for meaning in life, a mystical window onto the unconscious through which one could see the "raw materials of human mythology."[9] Certainly the experiences that the psychedelic drugs often produced—cosmic consciousness, heightened perception, universal fellow-feeling—seemed to many artists and intellectuals to connect naturally to Eastern religions, not unlike the way the effects of cosmetic Prozac tie into a Protestant ethic. But in at least one important way the attitudes toward the psychedelics current in the countercultural movements of the 1950s and 1960s differed from contemporary attitudes toward Prozac. Intellectuals and artists may well have seen psychedelics as a path to a more authentic life, but they also saw them as a means of revolt—as a way of transcending conventional ways of living. Perhaps Prozac can also be a tool of revolt (as Kramer says, by giving a person the energy to get up and do what needs to be done) but at least as often it seems to be a way of accommodating to conventional ways of life and making the best of them.

Lears sees a pattern in the American search for authenticity, especially in the calls from each generation, from the pre-World War I Greenwich Village intellectuals to the Beats, to throw off the repressive values of the generation preceding it. What has doomed this search to circularity in American life, argues Lears, is its lack of commitment to any wider values outside the self.[10] Whereas the search for a more authentic way of living was once fueled by religious or political concerns, it has gradually come to be motivated by purely internal goals, such as personal growth and psychic harmony. Without a wider framework of meaning, the search for authenticity eventually accommodates itself to the broader culture of consumer capitalism, and what begins as a generation's call for alternative values becomes a mere choice between "alternative lifestyles." For Lears, "What begins as discontent with a vapid modern culture ends as another quest for self-fulfillment—the dominant ideal of our sleeker, therapeutic culture." In a culture of consumer capitalism, this turn inward toward the self ultimately leads to barren territory. "As self-fulfillment and immediate gratification have become commodities on the mass market, calls for personal liberation have begun to ring hollow."[11]

Lears's diagnosis may be too harsh. Self-fulfillment as an ideal may seem excessively self-centered, but it can also be truly liberating—for example, in the case of women who previously had little opportunity for a career. Remember also that self-fulfillment is a *moral* ideal. That is, Americans generally do not see self-fulfillment as mere narcissism; they see a fulfilled life as a *higher* life, a better way to live out one's days. An unfulfilling life, a life that is not authentically yours, is not just an unhappy life, or a boring life, or even just a life of quiet desperation. It is a failure.

For the same reason, this ethic can also be oppressive. It is oppressive in that if you are unhappy or find life unfulfilling, there is something wrong with you, and not only should you pursue happiness, as our founding fathers have instructed us, you should pursue it aggressively. Why? Because if you don't you will be letting yourself down. You will be wasting the time you have on this earth. And if that means taking Prozac, so be it. In this way happiness is not just your right; it's your duty. This kind of thinking amounts to a kind of tyranny of happiness, which I think is especially pronounced in American life (I don't think a Scot, for example, would feel it nearly as strongly). It also gives cosmetic Prozac a kind of status here that it doesn't have elsewhere, and that we need to think more carefully about. If Prozac is seen as a kind of ticket to self-fulfillment, and self-fulfillment is your duty, then maybe we can begin to understand why Prozac has become so wildly popular among Americans.

## NOTES

1. Peter D. Kramer, *Listening to Prozac* (London: Fourth Estate Limited, 1994), p. 224.

2. Charles Taylor, "A Most Peculiar Institution," in *World, Mind and Ethics: Essays on the Ethical Philosophy of Bernard Williams,* ed. J.E.J. Altham and Ross Harrison (Cambridge: Cambridge University Press, 1995), p. 134.

3. See Charles Taylor's *Sources of the Self* (Cambridge, Massachusetts: Harvard University Press, 1989) and *The Malaise of Modernity* (Concord, Ontario: House of Anansi Press, 1991); and Lionel Trilling, *Sincerity and Authenticity* (Cambridge, Massachusetts: Harvard University Press, 1971).

4. Michael Walzer, *Thick and Thin: Moral Argument at Home and Abroad* (Notre Dame, Indiana: Notre Dame University Press, 1994).

**5.** Walker Percy, "The Man on the Train," in *The Message in the Bottle: How Queer Man Is, How Queer Language Is, and What One Has to Do with the Other* (New York: Farrar, Straus and Giroux, 1975).

**6.** T.J. Jackson Lears, *No Place of Grace: Antimodernism and the Transformation of American Culture, 1880–1920* (Chicago: University of Chicago Press, 1994).

**7.** See Lears, *No Place of Grace*, p. 75.

**8.** For an engaging history of the development of psychedelic drugs, see Jay Stevens, *Storming Heaven: LSD and the American Dream* (New York: Harper and Row, 1988).

**9.** Quoted in Stevens, *Storming Heaven*, p. 49.

**10.** Lears, *No Place of Grace*, p. 305–07.

**11.** Lears, *No Place of Grace*, p. 307.

SUSAN BORDO

# Braveheart, Babe, *and* the Contemporary Body

## Braveheart *and "Just Do It"*

I was stunned when Mel Gibson's *Braveheart* won the Oscar for best picture of the year. I know Hollywood loves a "sweeping" epic, and I liked the innovative use of mud and the absence of hairbrushes for the men (a commitment to material realism not matched in the commercial-perfect shots of the movie's heroines). But as interesting as it was to see Mel in unkempt cornrows, I didn't think it would add up to an Academy Award. Usually we require at least the semblance of an idea from our award winning epics. *Braveheart* is a one-liner (actually a one-worder)—and an overworked one. "Your heart is free. Have the courage to follow 'er," the young William Wallace is told by his father's ghost at the start of the film. And he does, leading an animal-house army of howling Scotsmen against the yoke of cruel and effete British tyrants. "Freedom!" he screams, as he is disemboweled in the concluding scene, refusing to declare allegiance to British rule. Between these two scenes, "free," "freedom," and "freemen" were intoned reverently or shrieked passionately. And that was about it for "content."

"Live free or die." That slogan does have historical and ideological resonance for Americans. But it's clearly not the collective fight against political tyranny that counts in the movie; it's the courage to act and the triumph of the undauntable, unconquerable action hero. Yes, Gibson makes William Wallace a fluent linguist, educated in Latin, well traveled, a man who uses his brain to plot battle strategy. But these traits are just a ploy to create the appearance of masculine stereotype busting. It's *doing*, not thinking, that reveals a man's worth in the film, whose notion of heroics is as toughguy as they come. In the last scene Wallace endures public stretching, racking, and evisceration so that Scotland will know he died without submitting, and Gibson (who directed the film as well as starred in it) makes the torture go on for a long, painful time. Wallace's resistance is really the point of the film. *Braveheart* has his eyes on a prize, and his will is so strong, so powerful, that he is able to endure anything to achieve it. The man has the right stuff.

This macho model of moral fortitude has a lot of living currency today—and for the first time, we now see it as applying to women as well as men. Undiluted testosterone drives *Braveheart*. Its band of Scottish rebels is described in a voice-over as fighting "like warrior-poets," an unmistakable nod to the mythopoetic men's movement to reclaim masculinity. King Longshank's son is a homosexual, and this detail is clearly coded in the film as signifying that he lacks the equipment to rule. But the movie's women, within the limits of their social roles, are as rebellious and brave-hearted as the men and enjoy watching a good fight. (In an early scene Wallace's girl's eyes light up as he and a fellow Scot have sport throwing bricks at each other's heads.) I think Gibson's idea of feminism is that one doesn't have to be male in order to be a real man—and it is an idea that is widely shared today, with "power" and "muscle" feminism as the culturally approved way of advancing the cause of women.

That women have just as much guts, willpower, and balls as men, that they can put their bodies through as much wear and tear, endure as much pain, and remain undaunted, was a major theme of the coverage of the 1996 Summer Olympics. Not since Leni Riefenstahl's Olympiad of 1936 has there been such a focus on the aesthetics of athletic perfection. But *this* version of beauty, like Riefenstahl's and like those stressed in the numerous photo-articles celebrating the Olympic body, has little to do with looking pretty. It's about strength, yes, and skill, but even more deeply it's about true grit. "Determined, defiant, dominating," the bold caption in the *New York Times Magazine* describes Gwen Torrence. (The same words, applied to rebellious wives or feminist politicos, have not been said so admiringly.) As in *Braveheart*, the ability to rise above the trials of the body is associated with the highest form of courage and commitment. Mary Ellen Clark's bouts of vertigo. Gail Devers's Graves' disease. Gwen Torrence's difficult childbirth. Amy Van Dyken's asthma. *Life* magazine describes these as personal tests of mettle sent by God to weed out the losers from the winners. And when gymnast Kerri Strug performed her second vault on torn tendons, bringing her team to victory in the face of what must have been excruciating pain, she became the unquestionable hero of the games (and set herself up with ten million dollars in endorsement contracts).

It's not the courage of these athletes I'm sniping at here; I admire them enormously. What bothers me is the message that is dramatized by the way we tell the tales of their success, a message communicated to us mortals too in commercials and ads. Nike has proven to be the master manipulator and metaphor maker in this game. Don't moan over life's problems or blame society for holding you back, Nike instructs us. Don't waste your time berating the "system." Get down to the gym, pick up those free weights, and turn things around. If it hurts, all the better. No pain, no gain. "Right after Bob Kempainen qualified for the marathon, he crossed the finish line and puked all over his Nike running shoes," Nike tells us in a recent advertisement. "We can't tell you how proud we were." A Nike commercial, shown during the games: "If you don't lose consciousness at the end, you could have run faster." Am I the only one who finds this recommendation horrifying in its implications? But consciousness apparently doesn't figure very much in our contemporary notions of heroism. What counts, as in *Braveheart*, is action. *Just Do It.* This is, of course, also what Nike wants us to do when we approach the cash register. (The call to act sends a disturbing political message as well. Movies like *Braveheart*, as a friend of mine remarked after we'd seen the film, seem designed to provide inspiration for the militia movement.)

The notion that all that is required to succeed in this culture is to stop whining, lace up your sneakers, and forge ahead, blasting your way through social limitations, personal tribulations, and even the laws of nature, is all around us. Commercials and advertisements egg us on: "Go for It!" "Know No Boundaries!" "Take Control!" Pump yourself up with our product—a car, a diet program, hair-coloring, sneakers— and take your destiny into your own hands. The world will open up for you like an oyster. Like the Sector watch advertisement (figure 1), AT&T urges us to "Imagine a world without limits" in a series of commercials shown during the 1996 Summer Olympics; one graphic depicts a young athlete polevaulting over the World Trade Center, another diving down an endless waterfall. And, indeed, in the world of these images there are no impediments—no genetic disorders, no body altering accidents, not even any fat—to slow down our progress to the top of the mountain. All that's needed is the power to *buy*.

The worst thing, in the *Braveheart*/Nike universe of values, is to be bossed around, told what to do. This independence creates a dilemma for advertisers, who somehow must convince hundreds of thousands of people to purchase the same product while assuring them that they

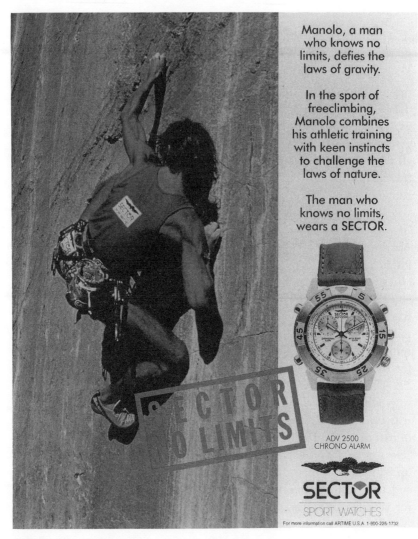

Manolo, a man who knows no limits, defies the laws of gravity.

In the sport of freeclimbing, Manolo combines his athletic training with keen instincts to challenge the laws of nature.

The man who knows no limits, wears a SECTOR.

ADV 2500
CHRONO ALARM

SECTOR
SPORT WATCHES
For more information call ARTIME U.S.A. 1-800-225-1732

**Figure 1.**   No limits.

are bold and innovative individualists in doing so. The dilemma is compounded because many of these products perform what Foucault and feminist theorists have called "normalization." That is, they function to screen out diversity and perpetuate social norms, often connected to race and gender. This screening happens not necessarily because advertisers are consciously trying to promote racism or sexism but because in order to sell products they have to either exploit or create a perception of personal lack in the consumer (who buys the product in the hope of filling that lack). An effective way to make the consumer feel inadequate is to take advantage of values that are already in place in the culture. For example, in a society where there is a dominant (and racialized) preference for blue-eyed blondes, there is a ready market for blue contact lenses and blonde hair-coloring. The catch is that ad campaigns promoting such products also reglamorize the beauty ideals themselves. Thus, they perpetuate racialized norms.

But people don't like to think that they are pawns of astute advertisers or even that they are responding to social norms. Women who have had or are contemplating cosmetic surgery consistently deny the influence of media images.[1] "I'm doing it for me," they insist. But it's hard to account for most of their choices (breast enlargement and liposuction being the most frequently performed operations) outside the context of current cultural norms. Surgeons help to encourage these mystifications. Plastic surgeon Barbara Hayden claims that breast augmentation today is "as individual as the patient herself"; a moment later in the same article another surgeon adds that the "huge 1980's look is out" and that many stars are trading their old gigantic breasts for the currently stylish smaller models![2]

*I'm doing it for me.* This saying has become the mantra of the television talk show, and I would gladly accept it if "for me" meant "in order to feel better about myself in this culture that has made me feel inadequate as I am." But people rarely mean this. Most often on these shows, the "for me" answer is produced in defiant refutation of some cultural "argument" (talk-show style, of course) on topics such as "Are Our Beauty Ideals Racist?" or "Are We Obsessed with Youth?" "No, I'm not having my nose (straightened)(narrowed) in order to look less ethnic. I'm doing it for me." "No, I haven't had my breasts enlarged to a 38D in order to be more attractive to men. I did it for me." In these constructions "me" is imagined as a pure and precious inner space, an "authentic" and personal reference point untouched by external values and demands. A place where we live free and won't be pushed around. It's the *Braveheart* place.

But we want both to imagine ourselves as bold, rebellious *Bravehearts* and to conform, to become what our culture values. Advertisers help us enormously in this self-deception by performing their own sleight-of-hand tricks with rhetoric and image, often invoking, as *Braveheart* does, the metaphor and hype of "political" resistance: "Now it's every woman's right to look good!" declares Pond's (for "age-defying" makeup). "What makes a woman revolutionary?" asks Revlon. "Not wearing makeup for a day!" answers a perfectly made-up Claudia Schiffer (quickly adding, "Just kidding, Revlon!"). A recent Gap ad: "The most defiant act is to be distinguished, singled out, marked. Put our jeans on." The absurdity of suggesting that everyone's donning the same (rather ordinary-looking) jeans can be a "defiant" and individualistic act is visually accompanied by two photos of female models with indistinguishable bodies.

## Power as Agency: Masking Reality

From evisceration at the hands of tyrants to defiance through dungarees may seem like a large leap. And in real terms, of course, it is. But we live in a world of commercial rhetoric that brooks no such distinctions. And not only commercial rhetoric. "Just Do It" is an ideology for our time, an idea that bridges the gulf between right and left, grunge and yuppie, chauvinist and feminist. The left wing didn't like "Just Say No," perhaps because it came from Nancy Reagan, perhaps because it was aimed at habits they didn't want to give up themselves. It isn't that easy, they insisted. The neighborhoods, the culture, social despair. . . . But the mind-over-matter message of "Just Do It," with its "neutral" origins (the brain of an ad woman) and associations with jogging, nice bodies, and muscle-lib for women, has roused no protests.

In a recent interview, rock star Courtney Love urged "liberals" to "breed" in order to outpopulate the Rush Limbaughs of the world. "It's not that hard," she said. "It's nine months. You know, just do it."[3] But right-wing ideologues like Limbaugh, who celebrate bootstrapping and Horatio Alger and scorn (what they view as) the liberal's creation of a culture of "victims," also advocate "just doing it."[4] And so too do celebrities like Oprah when they present themselves as proof that "anyone can make it if they want it badly enough and try hard enough." The implication here—which Oprah, I like to believe, would blanch at if she faced it squarely—is that if you don't succeed, it's proof that you didn't want it badly enough or try hard enough. Racism and sexism? Just so many hurdles to be jumped, personal challenges to be overcome. And what about the fact that in a competitive society someone always has to lose? We won't think about that, it's too much of a downer. Actually, in the coverage of the 1996 Olympics, everything short of "getting the gold" was constructed as losing. The men's 4 x 100 relay team, which won the silver medal, was interviewed by NBC after, as the commentator put it, their "defeat"! How can everyone be a winner if "winning" is reserved only for those who make it to the absolute pinnacle?

As far as women's issues go, "power feminists" are telling us that we're past all those tiresome harangues about "the beauty system" and "objectification" and "starving girls. " What's so bad about makeup, anyway? Isn't it my right to go for it? Do what I want with my body? Be all that I can be? Just a few years back "third-wave" feminist Naomi Wolf wrote a best-selling book, *The Beauty Myth* (1991), which spoke powerfully and engagingly to young women about a culture that teaches them they are nothing if they are not beautiful. But in a wink of the cultural zeitgeist, she declares in her latest, *Fire with Fire* (1993), that all that bitching and moaning has seen its day. Now, according to the rehabilitated Wolf, we're supposed to stop complaining and—you guessed it—"Just Do It." Wolf, in fact, offers Nike's commercial slogan as her symbol for the new feminism, which, as she describes it, is about "competition . . . victory . . . self-reliance . . . the desire to win."[5] Wolf is hardly alone in her celebratory mood. Betty Friedan has also said she is "sick of women wallowing in the victim state. We have empowered ourselves." A 1993 *Newsweek* article—most of its authors women—sniffs derisively at an installation of artist Sue Williams, who put a huge piece of plastic vomit on the floor of the Whitney Museum to protest the role of aesthetic ideals in encouraging the development of eating disorders. That kind of action once would have been seen as guerrilla theater. In 1993, *Newsweek* writers sneered: "Tell [the bulimics] to get some therapy and cut it out."[6]

Getting one's body in shape, of course, has become the exemplary practice, symbol, and means of empowerment in this culture. "You don't just shape your body," as Bally Fitness tells us. "You shape your life." As a manufacturer of athletic shoes, Nike—like Reebok and Bally—is dedicated to preserving the connection between having the right stuff and strenuous, physical activity. "It's about time," they declare disingenuously in a recent ad, "that the fitness craze that turned into the fashion craze that turned into the marketing craze turned back into the fitness craze." But despite Nike's emphasis on fitness, in contemporary commercial culture the rhetoric of taking charge of one's life has been yoked to everything from car purchases to hair-coloring, with physical effort and discipline often dropping out as a requirement. Even plastic surgery is continually described today—by patients, surgeons, and even by some feminist theorists—as an act of "taking control," "taking one's life into one's own hands" (a somewhat odd metaphor, under the circumstances).

These are the metaphors that dominate, for example, in sociologist Kathy Davis's arguments about cosmetic surgery and female "agency" in her *Reshaping the Female Body*. Among some academic feminists, an insistence on the efficacy of female "agency" is the more moderate, sober, scholarly sister of "power feminism." "Agency feminists" are not about to sing odes of praise to Nike, Reebok, or competition. They acknowledge that our choices are made within social and cultural contexts that are not all cause for celebration. But they do offer themselves as an alternative to what they caricature as the grim, petrified, politically dogmatic feminism of the past, now viewed as out of touch with the lives of real women. Those bad "old" feminists (I am one of these retrograde kvetchers, in some accounts) have a demeaning view of women as passive victims, tyrannized and suffocated by social norms, helpless pawns of social forces "beyond their control or comprehension." In contrast, the good, "new" feminism respects and honors the individual's choices as a locus of personal power, creativity, self-definition. So, for example, Davis argues that when a woman claims to have had her breasts enlarged "for herself," it's degrading and unsisterly not to accept this construction at face value. To deconstruct it—who is this "self"? where does it reside? in outer space? and where did it get the idea that it needed implants?—is to view the woman as a kind of helpless child who doesn't know her own mind and is not in charge of her own life. Contrasting herself to those feminists who view the industries in feminine self-improvement as "totalizing and pernicious" agents of women's oppression, Davis insists that these industries in fact play an important role in empowering women.

In a moment I will look more closely at Davis's arguments, which seem to me typical of a certain contemporary preference for the rhetoric of "agency" over close analysis of social context and cultural reality, a preference that mirrors—in more scholarly style, of course—the more popular images of empowerment I have been discussing. I will then talk about what aspects of reality these models of empowerment obscure. But first I'd like to note that arguments such as Davis's are often presented in the way she presents them—as an antidote against an imagined feminist position that holds that women are utterly passive and unconscious sponges, as subservient to cultural images as a browbeaten wife is to her abusive husband. Phrases like "cultural dope"— which are used to describe how the bad feminists allegedly view women—help vivify a nasty picture of condescending politicos who push women around with their theory as disdainfully as they claim the images do. Once such a picture is created, of course, the audience nods in agreement and approval, for the "new" feminism is sure to follow. But portraits of "victim feminists" are almost always caricatures. Davis, for example, accuses me of viewing women as "cultural dopes." But in fact where the power of cultural images is concerned, Davis and I actually have very little quarrel with each other. We both see cultural images as central elements in women's lives and we see them as contributing to a pedagogy of defect, in which women learn that various parts of their bodies are faulty, unacceptable. Neither of us views women as passive sponges in this process but (as I put it in my 1993 book *Unbearable Weight*) as engaged "in a process of making meaning, of 'labor on the body.' " We both recognize that there is ambiguity and contradiction, multiple meanings and consequences, in human motivations and choices.

While I object to Davis's placing the blame on feminists, I do have sympathy with Davis's desire to correct a general cultural tradition that has equated women with passivity rather than activity—the done to, not the doers, the acted upon, not the actors. But like many other attempts at "correcting" the mistakes of the past, Davis goes too far in the opposite direction. In this reaction we see a clear similarity between current academic obsessions with "agency" and the more popular versions of "power feminism," like Katie Roiphe's. Roiphe insists that most of what passes for "date rape" is actually an after-the-fact attempt on the part of young women to avoid responsibility for their own actions, like getting drunk on a date, for example. Roiphe, like academic "agency feminists," wants us to stop casting women as passive "victims," and she connects that perspective to the passe feminism of the past. But what Roiphe and Davis both seem to forget is that the main point of what is disparagingly (and misleadingly, I believe) called "victim feminism" was not to establish women's passivity or purity but to draw attention to the social and political context of personal behavior. Remember "The personal is the political"? Let's not forget that it wasn't so long ago that it was common coin to believe that women who get raped "ask for it" and that as far as beauty is concerned we are "our own worst enemies."

Where agency feminists and I most differ is over that magic word "agency." I don't see the word as adding very much beyond rhetorical cheerleading concerning how we, not the images, are "in charge" (the theory equivalent of "I did it for me"). More important, I believe that the cheering of "agency" creates a diversionary din that drowns out the real orchestra that is playing in the background, the consumer culture we live in and need to take responsibility for. To make this point clear, I need to look a bit more closely at Davis's arguments. Advertisements, fashion photos, cosmetic instructions, she points out (drawing on the work of eminent sociologist Dorothy Smith), all require "specialized knowledge" and "complex and skilled interpretive activities on the part of the female agent," who must "plan a course of action, making a series of on-the-spot calculations about whether the rigorous discipline required by the techniques of body improvement will actually improve her appearance given the specifics of her particular body."

By showing her how to correct various defects in her appearance ("Lose those unsightly bags under your eyes," "Turn your flabby rear-end into buns of steel," "Have a firm, sexy bosom for the first time in your life!" "Get a sexy stomach—fast!") the ads and instructions transform the woman into an agent of her own destiny, providing concrete objectives, goals, strategies, a plan of action. Davis quotes Smith here: "The text instructs her [the woman] that her breasts are too small/too big; she reads of a remedy; her too small breasts become remediable. She enters into the discursive organization of desire; now she has an objective where before she had only a defect."[7] So the "sexy stomach" article (just one example of the scores of fitness features that appear regularly in women's magazines; see figure 2) addresses a consumer whose stomach, the text implies, is not yet sexy; at the same time, the lean body of the model offers visual "proof" to all but the fittest readers that they are indeed in less than ideal shape "for bikini weather." But it's not too late, we are reassured; those abs can still be whipped into shape with the right exercises. This prescription for improvement, as Davis would interpret it, allows the woman to take control of her own body in a way that was unavailable to her before she read the article.

Now, just so you know that I'm not really some sour old "victim feminist," let me say at once that make-up and fashion can be creative fun, and I enjoy exchanging beauty tips with my friends. But Davis is claiming more—that it is precisely the learning to see ourselves as defective and lacking, needful of improvement and remedy (too fat, too flat-chested, too dark-skinned, too wrinkled), that mobilizes us, puts us in charge of our lives! Is this argument not strained, if not downright perverse? I know that Davis views what she is doing as correcting the sins of other feminists, who, as she describes them, are so focused on the "tyranny" of the big bad beauty system that they don't notice the female subjects who are participating in it. But her

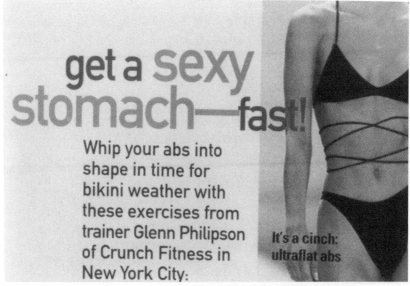

**Figure 2.** Be an agent. Whip those abs!

critique goes beyond regarding women as subjects to equating the self-scrutinizing subjectivity these ads encourage with a state of liberation. In the quote from Smith, just when is the woman in question supposed to have been in her disempowered "before" state, when she "only had a defect" without an objective? Before she read the liberating "text" that tells her how to remedy her too small breasts or insufficiently flat stomach? In telling her how to remedy this "defect" is the text not simply providing a cure (at a price, of course—they are selling something here, let's not forget) for the very poison it has administered?

To see this point more concretely, consider this ad (I have chosen one from another cultural period, situated within notions of femininity that emphasize delicacy and fragility, in order to encourage a bit of distance): "Conspicuous Nose Pores: How to Reduce Them" (figure 3). The formula here is exactly as Davis describes it. First we are warned that "complexions otherwise flawless are often ruined by conspicuous nose pores." The ad goes on to describe with great specificity and detail the beauty regime that will correct those conspicuous nose pores. As Davis would interpret this ad, the specification of such a regime makes the "female agent the *sine qua non* of the feminine beauty system." By telling women what they need to *do* in order to bring their bodies up

200   *Susan Bordo*

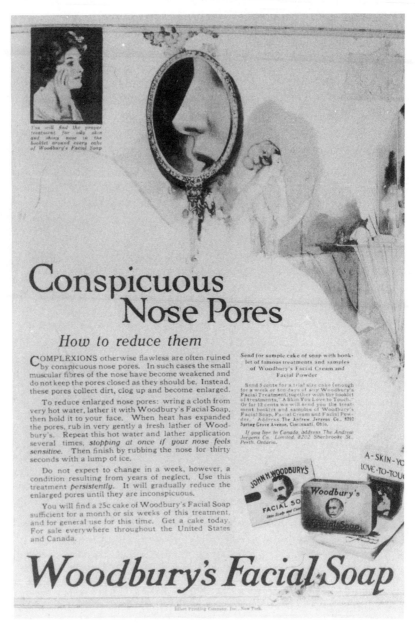

**Figure 3.**   Ruined by conspicuous nose pores.

to par (defined here, I want to note, as "flawless"—a goal that will keep female agents busy till they topple into the grave, perfectly embalmed), they inspire women to no longer suffer their dissatisfaction passively, impotently, but as "an active process." "Rather than immobilizing women, bodily imperfections provide the opportunity for action."

But what made the woman with the conspicuous nose poses dissatisfied to begin with? What gave her the idea that they were "ruinous" to her beauty? Probably not this ad alone. But certainly this ad, among other social factors, creates the very condition of perceived defect that it now tells women how to overcome. By this logic it would be a sorry day indeed if women were to become content with the way they look. Without all those defects to correct we would lose an important arena for the enactment of our creative agency! There doesn't seem to be much chance of that happening though. Instead, the sites of defect have multiplied for women, and men increasingly have been given more of these wonderful opportunities for agency, too, as magazines and products devoted to the enhancement and "correction" of their appearance have multiplied.

I have spent so much time on this point not to whip the agency feminist position to its knees but because what is obscured in Davis's discussion of ads and beauty features is exactly what must be kept at the forefront of any cultural analysis of practices of bodily improvement. There is a consumer system operating here that depends on our perceiving ourselves as defective and that will continually find new ways to do this. That system—and others connected to it, generating new technologies and areas of expertise organized around the diagnosis and correction of "defect"—is masked by the rhetoric of personal empowerment.

Take cosmetic surgery, which Davis describes as an empowering "solution" to an individual's problems with body image, a way for women to actively "take control" of their bodies and "take the reins" of their lives "in hand." (Ads for cosmetic surgery, by the way, use the exact same argument.) Davis supports her position by drawing on interviews with a handful of individual women, whose "defects" range from facial deformity to too small breasts and who all describe surgery as having helped them. I am disturbed, to begin with, by Davis's failure to draw distinctions between *kinds* of body alteration. Cosmetic surgery covers an enormous range of corrections, from the repair of major birth defects to Roseanne's cheek implants to Liz's liposuction. But for Davis all women's body-image problems are given the same weight, and they are represented by her in terms such as "terrible suffering" and "valiant struggle." I don't deny that many of us in this culture have deep wounds of shame about our bodies (I certainly do); I have written extensively about this, I believe with empathy and understanding. But there are still distinctions to be drawn here, distinctions that are rapidly disappearing in our talk-show culture, where everyone's story is worth a show and is sensationalized on the air as dramatically as possible.

By treating breast augmentations and operations to correct facial deformities as the same by virtue of their ability to "empower" individuals, we lose the ability to critique the former from a cultural point of view. I don't have a problem with the notion that an individual's long and fruitless struggle to live with a particular "defect" may end happily when that defect is corrected. But assessing "the dilemma of cosmetic surgery" (as Davis calls it) requires more than taking these individual snapshots of satisfied customers (or dissatisfied ones, for that matter). We need a picture of the landscape, too. For cosmetic surgery is more than an individual choice; it is a burgeoning industry and an increasingly normative cultural practice. As such, it is a significant contributory cause of women's suffering by continually upping the ante on what counts as an acceptable face and body. In focusing on narratives of individual "empowerment," Davis—like Oprah's guests who claim they did it "for themselves"—overlooks the fact that the norms that encouraged these individuals to see themselves as defective are enmeshed in the practice and institution of cosmetic surgery itself. And so is individual behavior.

I now want to sharpen my focus to discuss some of the cultural and institutional aspects of cosmetic surgery that are missing from Davis's stories of individual empowerment. Let me say, as a general introduction to this discussion, that we have barely begun to confront— and are not yet in a position to adequately assess—the potential cultural consequences of regarding the body as "cultural plastic,"[8] to be deconstructed and rearranged as we desire. For this reason alone, we need to keep track of cultural trends, not just personal narratives. Our relationship to our bodies has clearly become more and more an investment in them as "product" and image, requiring alteration as fashions change. Consider breast augmentation, now increasingly widespread, and its role in establishing new norms against which smaller or less firm breasts are seen as *defective*. Micromastia is the clinical term, among plastic surgeons, for "too small" breasts. Such "disorders" are, of course, entirely aesthetic and completely socially "constructed." Anyone who doubts this should recall the 1920s, when women were binding their breasts to look more boyish. Today, with artificial implants the norm among movie stars and models, an adolescent boy who has grown up learning what a woman's body looks like from movies, cable television, and magazines may wonder what's wrong when his girlfriend lies down and her breasts flop off to the side instead of standing straight up in the air. Will we soon see a clinical term for "too floppy" breasts?

As the augmented breast becomes the norm, the decision to have one's breasts surgically enhanced becomes what the psychiatrist Peter Kramer has called "free choice under pressure." We can choose not to have such surgery. No one is holding a gun to our heads. But those who don't—for example, those who cannot afford the surgery—are at an increasingly significant professional and personal disadvantage. The same is true of facelifts and other surgeries to "correct" aging, which are also becoming more normative. More and more of my friends— these are teachers, therapists, writers, not movie stars and models— are contemplating or even planning surgery. We scan our faces every morning for signs of downward drift, and we measure our decline against the lifted and tightened norms of the images that surround us. For me, viewing the Academy Awards was something of an exercise in self-flagellation, as actresses my own age and older stepped up to the podium, each one looking younger and tighter around the eyes than she had ten years ago. At forty-nine I have come to feel each fresh capitulation to surgery on the part of these actresses as a personal affront; my own face, after all, will be judged by the standards that these actresses are establishing. As a teacher and writer, my status and success depend far less on my looks than they do for other women. If it all gets to me, imagine how women feel in the countless service and public relations positions for which youthful looks are a job prerequisite.

The fact is that the plastically reconstructed and preserved faces and bodies of the forty- and fifty-something actresses who came of age with us have made the ideal of aging beautifully and "gracefully" obsolete. Now we are supposed to "defy" our age, as Melanie Griffith (her own lips decidedly poutier than they were a few years ago) instructs us in her commercials for Revlon. In thinking about this "defiance" of age, I often wonder what existential traumas lie in store for those who have not been slowly acclimated to the decline of their bodies, learning to accept and accommodate the small changes that happen gradually over the years, but who have become habituated instead to seeing those changes as an occasion for immediate action. Although for now true "scalpel slaves" are generally found only among the fairly wealthy, first surgeries are becoming more and more common among people of all classes, races, and ages.[9] (We should know by now how such practices tend to "trickle down" in this culture.[10]) And first surgeries often lead to more. Some surgeons acknowledge that once you begin "correcting" for age, it's all too easy to start sliding down the slope of habituation. "Plastic surgery sharpens your eyesight," says one. "You get something done, suddenly you're looking in the mirror every five minutes—at imperfections nobody else can see."[11]

The pressure to have age-defying surgery is now creeping across the gender gap too. Men used to be relatively exempt from the requirement to look young; gray hair and wrinkles were (and still mostly are) a code for experience, maturity, and wisdom. But in a "Just Do It" culture that now equates youth and fitness with energy and competence—the "right stuff"—fortyish businessmen are feeling increasing pressure to dye their hair, get liposuction on their spare tires, and have face-lifts in order to compete with younger, fitter-looking men and women. In 1980, men accounted for only 10 percent of plastic surgery patients. In 1994 they were 26 percent.[12] These numbers will undoubtedly rise, as plastic surgeons develop specialized angles to attract men ("penile enhancement" is now advertised in the sports sections of major newspapers) and disinfect surgery of its associations with feminine vanity. Also thanks to the efforts of surgeons, who now argue that one should start "preventive" procedures while the skin is still elastic, younger and younger people are having surgery. Here is the text of an advertisement I came across recently in the local (Lexington, Kentucky) paper:

> Picture this scenario. You're between the ages of thirty-five and fifty. You feel like you are just hitting your stride. But the face in the mirror is sending out a different message. Your morning facial puffiness hangs around all day. You're beginning to resemble your parents at a point when they began looking old to you. If you prefer a more harmonic relationship between your self-perception and outer image, you may prefer to tackle these concerns before they become too obvious. You may benefit from a face-lift performed at an earlier age. There is no carved-in-stone perfect time or age to undergo a face-lift. For those who place a high priority on maintaining a youthful appearance, any visual disharmony between body and soul can be tackled earlier when cosmetic surgical goals tend to be less aggressive and it is easier to obtain more natural-looking results. The reason is: Younger skin and tissues have more elasticity so smoothness can be achieved with surgery.

What this ad obscures is that the "disharmonies" between body and soul that thirty-five- and forty-year-old (!) women may be experiencing are not "carved-in-stone" either but are in large part the product of our *cultural* horror of wrinkles and lines—a horror, of course, that surgeons are fueling. Why should a few lines around our eyes be experienced as "disharmonious" with the energy and vitality that we feel "inside," unless they are coded as a sign of decrepitude (looking like our parents—good heavens, what a fate!). That these lines can be coded otherwise is a theme of a Murad ad (see figure 4). But while Dr. Murad acknowledges that our various lines and wrinkles are markers of the accumulated experience and accomplishment of our lives, the ad recommends that we wipe our faces clean of them. This ad, like many others, attempts to have its commercial cake without having to "eat" criticism along with it, to value "character" (along with critics of the beauty system) while insisting that it doesn't have to show on our faces (just buy our product).

The woman in the ad is dazzling, of course; but that only serves as a reminder of just how fragile beauty is, and how important it is to start protecting it against age before time gets the upper hand. We are now being encouraged to view this aging process as a disaster for our sense of "who we really are" (our "self," our "soul," as the ad puts it) and as a slippery slope heading for the time when we will be utterly beyond saving, social detritus. (A fifty-nine-year-old face-lift patient describes the skin around her neck as "garbage old, ugly, sagging . . . garbage."[13]) We are always holding our finger in that dam, getting in as much "life" as we can before the deluge, as though "life" ends when we are no longer young and firm. If we thought of the "real self" as evolving into new and unpredictable forms (perhaps with "harmonies" in store that are deeper and more satisfying than looking good), we might look on wrinkles and lines as an opportunity to engage in a learning process about the inevitability of change, the impermanence of all things. Yes, and about our own physical vulnerability, and mortality. Others around us are dying too. Focusing on unsightly wrinkles and disfiguring nose pores, we don't have to look at that.

Every "correction" of aging represents a lost opportunity to do this important psychological work. And if cosmetic surgery becomes the normalized, affordable alternative that it now seems to be becoming, how will generations used to "correcting" their bodies surgically according to perfected norms cope with the inevitable failure of such correction? For, you know, you just can't go on doing it forever. For those

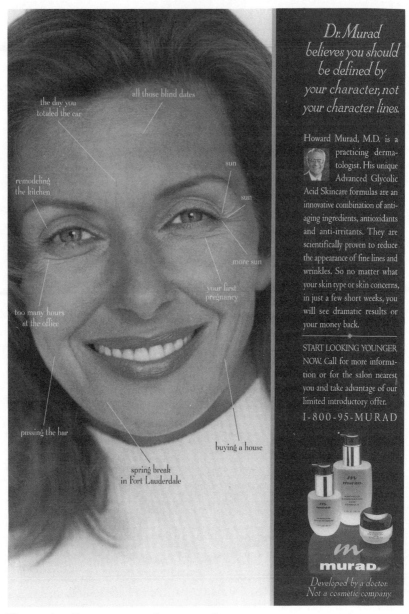

**Figure 4.**   Erase your age from your face.

who try, the stretched and staring, often cadaverous mask of plastically preserved beauty becomes itself a marker of age and impending death. This transformation is partly why I am not inclined to surgery. I would rather get used to aging gradually, to changes in the way I am seen by others, to the inevitability of frailty creeping into my presence and mode of being in the world, to my own mortality, so that I can be prepared and respond consciously and with dignity and, yes, in a way that I hope will actually enhance my physical appearance. I care about looks (I don't live on Uranus, after all). But I'd rather be a vibrant old woman than embalm myself in a mask of perpetual youth.

In assessing the consequences of our burgeoning surgical culture, there are ethical and social as well as existential issues to be confronted. As I noted in *Unbearable Weight,* the surgeries that people "choose" often assimilate ethnic and racial features to a more "white" norm. "Does anyone in this culture," I asked, "have his or her nose reshaped to look more 'African' or 'Jewish'?" The answer, of course, is no. Given our history of racism—a history in which bodies that look "too black" or obviously Jewish have been refused admittance to public places and even marked for death—how can we regard these choices as merely "individual preferences"? In Japan it has become increasingly common for job-seeking female college graduates to have their eyes surgically altered to appear more occidental. Such a "Western" appearance, it is widely acknowledged, gives a woman the edge in job interviews. But capitulating to this requirement—although it may be highly understandable from the point of view of the individual's economic survival and advancement—is to participate in a process of racial normalization and to make it harder for others to refuse to participate. The more established the new norm, the higher the costs of resisting—"free choice under pressure." The same points can be made about many of the operations that people have performed on them in this country. And while some might celebrate being able to "choose" one's features as part of a "melting pot" society, as eradicating racial differences that we don't need and that have only caused pain and suffering, we should face the fact that only certain ingredients in the pot are being encouraged to "melt" here.

Situating "personal" choices in social, cultural, and economic contexts such as these raises certain issues for the thoughtful individual, one being the interpretation of his or her own situation, which becomes harder to see as a "free," autonomous choice done "for oneself"; another being his or her complicity in the perpetuation of racialized norms *and* in the suffering of other people. These issues of complicity may be most striking in the case of influential and highly visible culture makers such as Cher and Madonna—who never take any responsibility for the images they create, of course. But those of us who aren't celebrities also influence the lives we touch. Mothers (and fathers) set standards for their children, sisters and brothers for their siblings, teachers for their students, friends for their friends. Adult behavior reinforces cultural messages sent to teens and preteens about the importance of looking good, of fitting in—pressures that young people then impose, often brutally, on one another. (One of my students wrote that the images of slenderness only began to "get to her" when she realized that her parents also "believed in them.")

Not that many years ago parents who smoked never thought twice about the instructional effect this might be having on their children, in legitimating smoking, making it seem adult and empowering. A cultural perspective on augmentation, face-lifts, cosmetic "ethnic cleansing" of Jewish and black noses, Asian eyes, and so on similarly might make parents think twice about the messages they are sending their children, might make them less comfortable with viewing their decisions as purely "personal" or "individual" ones. And they should think twice. We are all culture makers as well as culture consumers, and if we wish to be considered "agents" in our lives—and have it mean more than just a titular honor—we need to take responsibility for that role.

To act consciously and responsibly means understanding the culture we live in, even if it requires acknowledging that we are not always "in charge." That we are not always in charge does not mean that we are "dopes." In fact, I think the really dopey thing is living with the illusion that we are "in control," just because some commercial (or ad for surgery) tells us so. In the culture we live in, individuals are caught between two contradictory injunctions. On the one hand, an ideology of triumphant individualism and mind-over-matter heroism urges us to "Just Do It" and tries to convince us that we can "just do it," whatever our sex, race, or circumstances. This is a mystification. We are not runners on a level field but on one that is pocked with historical inequities that make it much harder for some folks to lace up their Nikes and speed to the finish line—until the lane in which they are running has been made less rocky and the hidden mines excavated and removed. A few of us, if we are very, very lucky (circumstances still do count, willpower isn't everything, despite what the commercials tell us), do have our moments of triumph. But it is often after years of struggle in which we have drawn on many resources other than our own talent, resolve, and courage. We have been helped by our friends and our communities, by social movements, legal and political reform, and sheer good fortune. And many, of course, don't make it.

But on the other hand, while consumerism assures us that we can (and should) "just do it," it continually sends the contradictory message that we are defective, lacking, inadequate. This message is the missing context of the stories of empowerment that Davis tells, rewriting the "old" feminist scripts. But what she leaves out just happens to be the very essence of advertising and the fuel of consumer capitalism, which cannot allow equilibrium or stasis in human desire. Thus, we are not permitted to feel satisfied with ourselves and we are "empowered" only and always through fantasies of what we *could* be.

This is not a plot; it's just the way the system works. Capitalism adores proliferation and excess; it abhors moderation. One moment the culture begins talking about greater health consciousness, which is surely a good thing that no one would deny. But the next moment we've got commercials on at every hour for every imaginable exercise and diet product, and people are spending huge quantities of their time trying to achieve a level of "fitness" that goes way beyond health and straight into obsession. Technological possibilities emerge that allow surgeons to make corrective repairs of serious facial conditions; before long our surgeons have become Pygmalions of total self-transformation, advertising the slightest deviation from the cultural "norm" as a problem needing to be solved, an impediment to happiness (as in the ad in figure 5). Drugs like Prozac are developed to treat serious clinical depressions: the next moment college clinics are dispensing these pills to help students with test anxiety.

The multiplication of human "defect" is aided by factors other than economic. Drug companies may be focused on profits, but those folks at the university clinic are genuinely concerned about students and want to make their lives easier. Cosmetic surgeons, while fabulously paid, are rarely in it for the money alone. Often, they are carried to excess not by dreams of yachts but by savior fantasies and by pure excitement about the technological possibilities. Nowadays, those possibilities can be pretty fantastic, as fat is suctioned from thighs and injected into lips, breast implants inserted through the bellybutton, penises enlarged through "phalloplasty," and nipples repositioned. Each of us, working in our own professional niche, is focused on the possibilities for our

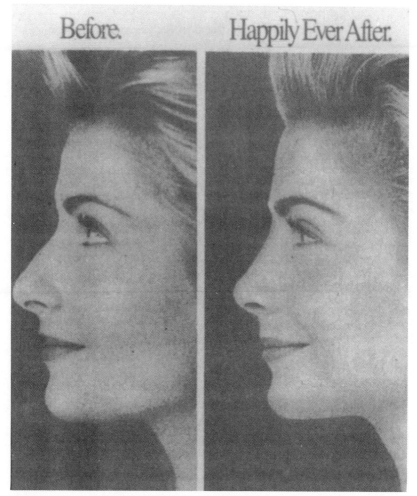

**Figure 5.** Normalizing noses.

own "agency" and personal effectiveness working within that niche, so we rarely stand back to survey the big picture. That's precisely why we need cultural criticism.

Recently I had a personal experience that brought freshly home to me the central and complex role the multiplication of "defect" plays in our culture and the way it can be masked by a rhetoric of agency. With a very specific request, I went to a dentist specializing in cosmetic dentistry. Because of antibiotics I had been given in infancy, my front teeth were starting to darken and I wanted to have them capped. I described the problem to the dentist and he asked me to smile. No problem with capping the teeth, he said. But wouldn't I also like a less gummy smile and a correction of my overbite? I told him that I thought I had a pretty nice smile as it was. He was stone silent. I was somewhat hurt, even shaken by his refusal to reassure me, and suddenly old childhood insecurities began to surface. At the age of eight I was convinced that I looked like Alfred E. Neuman, from Mad magazine. On better days I saw a small, freckled, overweight rabbit in the mirror. I had thought those days were long gone, but now I was looking again in the mirror for signs that "What, Me Worry?" Neuman or chubby Bugs was really still lurking there. Letty Cottin Pogrebin, in her new book on aging, describes a similar experience at her dermatologist:

> It started with a small cyst on my back and two bumps, each the size of a lemon pit, on my thigh. For no apparent reason, my skin occasionally produces these outcroppings—my friend Gale calls them the "barnacles of age"—and, given the gaping hole in the ozone layer and the idiosyncrasies of skin cancer, I've learned to take it seriously. Off I went to the dermatologist, who performed minor surgery on the lemon pits and, to my relief, pronounced the bumps benign. At the end of the checkup, the doctor glanced at my face, then at my chart, then again at my face. "You look pretty good for your age," he declared. "But you'd look a hundred percent better without those fat pouches under your eyes."[14]

Pogrebin then goes on to describe in fresh and honest detail her own ambivalence about the possibility of surgery (she decided against it). She does not, however, comment further on the role her doctor played, not just in normalizing surgery in her eyes but in suggesting that she was an appropriate candidate for it—when she had come in on an entirely different matter. When people claim to be having surgery "for themselves," they frequently mean that they are not being urged to do so by husbands or boyfriends. But husbands and boyfriends are not the only eyes that survey and evaluate women; the gaze of the doctor, especially with the tremendous authority that doctors have in this culture, may hold a lot of weight, may even be experienced as the discerning point of view of a generalized cultural observer, an "objective" assessor of defect. Writing for *New York* magazine, a twenty-eight-year-old, 5 foot 6, 118-pound Lily Burana describes how a series of interviews with plastic surgeons—the majority of whom had recommended rhinoplasty, lip augmentation, implants, liposuction, and eyelid work—changed her perception of herself from "a hardy young sapling that could do with some pruning . . . to a gnarled thing that begs to be torn down to the root and rebuilt limb by limb."[15]

Under these cultural conditions the desire to be "normal" or "ordinary," which Kathy Davis claims is the motivation for most cosmetic surgeries, is much more slippery than she makes it out to be. Davis makes the point that none of her subjects describe their surgeries as having been done for the sake of "beauty" but insist they only wanted to feel "ordinary." But in a culture that proliferates defect and in which the surgically perfected body ("perfect" according to certain standards, of course) has become the model of the "normal," even the ordinary body becomes the defective body. This continual upping of the ante of physical acceptability is cloaked by ads and features that represent the cosmetic surgeon as a blessed savior, offering miraculous technology to end long-standing pain. The "Before/Happily Ever After" noted earlier ("She didn't like her nose. She felt it kept her from looking and feeling her best.") offers its advice to an imagined consumer who is already troubled and ashamed of her defect. An unhappy reader is also assumed in "Correcting a Gummy Smile" (figure 6): "Do you hold back when you smile so as not to reveal too much gum? If you've always hated your smile and tried to hide it, you'll learn how a simple plastic surgery procedure . . ."). But how many women who are basically

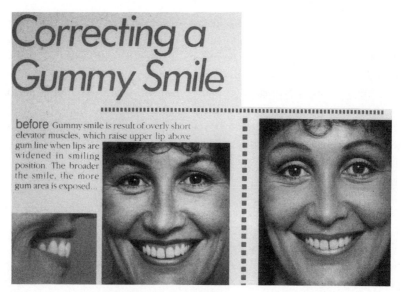

**Figure 6.** The shame of a gummy smile.

satisfied with their appearance begin to question their self image on the basis of images and advice presented in these features or—even more authoritatively—dispensed to them by their doctors? As noted, the "gumminess" of my own smile was of no concern to me until after I had seen the dentist; but under his care I began to wonder if it wasn't in actuality something I'd better hide . . . or "correct."

The spell was broken, however, when a few days after my appointment I received a computer-generated set of recommendations from the same dentist. The recommendations were phrased so as to make his prescribed course of cosmetic alteration seem precisely individualized and entirely a matter of satisfying my stated desires. My name was plugged in, of course, and the recommendations chosen from a set list of options, ready to be inserted with a keystroke, each with its own little prefabricated paragraph. The pretense that it was written specially for me didn't bother me too much (we are used to this nowadays), but I became enraged when I saw that he had inserted all the options that were his idea as though they represented my expressed dissatisfactions and desires. It went something like this: "Susan Bordo: You have taken an important step toward giving yourself a beautiful, youthful smile. You have told us that you are dissatisfied with the discoloration in your teeth, with the gumminess of your smile, that you would like a shorter, neater bite, and a brighter, younger look." The recommendations that followed would have cost me about $25,000 to implement.

I realized while going over this form that no patient was going to get away without at least one or two of those prefabricated keystrokes. "Gummy smile." "Shorter bite." And so forth. If you are trained to see defect, you will. I went for a second opinion, from a family dentist, and I was relieved to hear that she thought my smile was fine as it was and that there was no need to cut huge trenches in my gums in order to make me look more like Michelle Pfeiffer. I never called the first dentist back, but a few days later I received a message on my answering machine in which he wondered why I had not come back. He had wanted so much, he said, to give me the nice smile I wanted.

## Babe: *A Real Metaphor in our Lives*

Freedom. Choice. Autonomy. Self. Agency. These are powerful words in our culture, fighting words. But they are also words that are increasingly empty in many people's experience. Are we invoking the rhetoric with such desperation precisely because the felt reality is slipping away, running through our fingers? I think about the pain and self-doubt, the compulsions and disorders that often accompany our efforts at becoming what the culture rewards—particularly among my students, so many of whom have serious problems with food, weight, and body image. Then I listen to the rousing cries of "power feminism" in both its commercial and its academic formulations: "Just Do It!" "Take Control!" "Go for It!" There is a discordance for me between the celebration of "agency" and empowerment and what I see going on in people's lives today.

Don't misunderstand me here. I think that there have been great gains in the status of women in this culture. And I love seeing women with muscles, particularly when they project strength and solidity—as they did on the bodies of some of the Olympic runners, swimmers, ball players—and not merely a tighter, toned, anorexic aesthetic. I'm thrilled to see women who don't feel they need to hold back on their skill and power in order to remain "feminine." But let us not be deceived into believing, along with the magazine articles and TV commentaries, that we are at the dawn of a new, "postfeminist" age for women.

Do we really think that the twelve-year-old who becomes obsessed with looking like Gabriel Reece is really in *such* an alternative universe to the one who wants to look like Kate Moss? Sure, rigorous weight training is probably less dangerous and makes you feel better than compulsive dieting (although my students seem perfectly capable of combining the two in a double-punishing daily regime). But isn't the real problem here the tyrannized relation in which young women stand to these images (whatever they may be), their sense that they personally are of no use, no value, ugly, unacceptable, without a future, unless they can get their bodies into the prescribed shape? How can feature writer Holly Brubach of the *New York Times* look around her—at the eating disorders, the exercise compulsions, the self-scrutiny and self-flagellation of young women today—and honestly write that "women, as they have gradually come into their own, have at last begun to feel at home in their bodies"?[16] Call me a "victim feminist," but I just don't see it.

The triumphs that we wrest from those arenas of bodily improvement in which we are all supposed to be able to "just do it" are especially tenuous, reflecting the more generally unstable and desperate quality of life today. Both literally and figuratively there is an on-the-treadmill quality to the lives of most women (and men) as we struggle to achieve some sort of homeostasis in a culture that doesn't really want that from us. The practices of dieting and exercise succinctly capture this treadmill quality. Dieting, it has now been fairly decisively established, is self-defeating and self-perpetuating, for physiological as well as psychological reasons. Our bodies, thinking we are starving, slow down their metabolism and make it harder for us to burn up the few calories we are eating. Feelings of deprivation (especially combined with the demoralization of working hard at a diet and not getting very far) lead to bingeing, which leads to a sense of failure and hopelessness, and so more bingeing. Even the "successful" diet that results in the desired weight loss is a tenuous achievement. While dieting, pumped up with excitement over the project of "taking control," imagining our gorgeous bodies-to-be, we may be able to live (in hope, if not contentment) on broccoli and fat-free cheese. But once we reach our goal, this regime is no longer part of a project with a clear beginning and end. It's a life sentence. The "Healthy Choice" dinners stare at us: "This is how it's gonna be from now on, baby. Get used to it!" Most of us, understandably, don't feel we can.

Nowadays they tell us that the way to beat the diet syndrome is to exercise. So, many of us exercise in order to be able to eat. I have friends who use the StairMaster like a purge; after a big meal, they hop on it. The oddness of this practice notwithstanding, exercise can of course be healthy, stress-relieving, and empowering. It can also become a compulsive daily ritual around which people organize and subordinate all other activities, and frankly I've found this compulsiveness to be more common than not. I have friends and students who become intensely anxious when they miss just one day at the gym, who view their daily routines not as maintaining health or fitness but as a kind of finger-in-the-dam against disaster. I don't see this as paranoia but as a recognition of the reality that something in them is always near rebellion against the struggle to simply maintain the status quo. That rebellious little imp—the imp that wants to "let go" instead of stay in control—can't be let out of the bottle, ever. He's too dangerous.

I have serious problems with any theory, rhetoric, or narrative that masks these realities in favor of the inspiring (but inevitably deceptive) "success story" that, like the commercials and ads, captures a moment of "empowerment" and makes it stand for the reality of things. And so I come to *Babe*, which did not win the Academy Award but which moved and haunted me for weeks after I saw it. For a long time I tried to put my finger on just why that was. As I've said, I generally bristle against the triumphant success story. And *Babe*, like *Braveheart* (and

*Rocky*), is a success story, a tale of individual empowerment and personal triumph against enormous odds, of questing, self-transformation, and, you might even say, transcendence of the body. A little pig, seemingly destined to be dinner, dreams of becoming a sheepdog—and he succeeds! Crowds cheer and tears flow. And so did mine (dry at the end of *Braveheart* and *Rocky*).

When I tried to explain to a more cynical friend why I loved the film, I grasped impotently at the available takes on the film then circulating in magazines and among intellectuals. "Allegory of social prejudice," that sort of thing. But I knew that wasn't exactly what did it for me, and when my friend pressed on, amazed that I could be so taken by what she saw as a sentimental fantasy, I realized that sentimental—in the sense of wrenching emotion while falsifying reality—was precisely what I found *Babe* not to be and a large part of why it moved me so powerfully. *Braveheart*, apparently based on real events, seemed like a slick commercial to me from start to finish. But *Babe*—a fable with talking animals— was for me a moment of reality in a culture dominated by fantasy.

*Babe*, on the face of it, seems far removed from the land of StairMasters, liposuction, and face-lifts—and it is certainly nothing like a Nike commercial. *Babe*'s personal triumph takes place in a world that—as the film never lets us forget—permits such moments only for a very few. On the farm most of the animals eke their joy humbly from the circumscribed routines and roles allotted to them—and they are the lucky ones, the safe ones. The others—those who are destined to be eaten—tremble on little islands of temporary peace, the vulnerability and perishability of their existence always hovering before them. Death for them will not be accompanied by the dignifying hoopla of the big battle or the knowledge that they have made a statement for history. They will have no control over when death comes, and they will be unable to make the "why" of it more meaningful than the fact that others are luckier and more powerful and more arrogant than they are. Theirs is a world in which those who can "just do it" are a privileged few. A world in which "agency" is real but limited and "empowerment" possible but hardly an everyday affair. A world in which the notion that we are "in charge," "in control," "at the reins" is strictly an illusion. Existence is precarious for the animals on the farm, as it is materially for many people, and as it is existentially for all of us, whether we recognize it or not. We can try to avoid this recognition with illusions of "agency," fantasies of staying young forever, and the distractions of "self-improvement," but it only lies in wait for us.

It is very important to the emotional truth of the film that *Babe* himself learns about the fragility of his safety. When he decides to go on anyway, it is not as a hopeful hero-to-be, dreaming of glory, but out of the simple fact that despite "the way things are" in the awful world he has learned about, there is still the unanswerable, unbreakable bond between him and the Boss. The men in *Braveheart* are bonded too. But, as Gibson directs it, the relationship amounts to a fraternity handshake, a pledge of affiliation; they're all pumped up, looking out over the grandeur of the countryside, ready to take up arms together. The bond between *Babe* and the Boss is established in a very different sort of exchange, in which each, in a Kierkegaardian leap of faith, bravely lets down his defenses in a moment of simple caring for and trust in the other. The taciturn and reserved farmer, trying to get depressed *Babe* to eat and obeying some wild impulse of inspiration, leaps up and performs an unrestrained, goofy hornpipe for him. *Babe* watches and, although he has heard "the way things are" from Fly, his surrogate-mother (pigs get eaten, even by the Boss and his wife), cedes final authority to the reasons of the heart. He eats.

*Babe*'s world is the one we live in; heroic moments are temporary and connections with others are finally what sustain us. It is a reality we may be inclined to forget as we try to create personal scenarios that will feel like Olympic triumphs and give us the power and "agency" over our bodies and lives that the commercials promise. But we still feel the emotional tug of abandoned dreams of connection and intimacy and relationships that will feed us in the open-hearted way that the Boss feeds little *Babe* and *Babe*'s eating feeds him. My cynical friend disliked the movie for—as she saw it—idealizing parent-child relations through scenes such as this (and *Babe*'s relationship with his surrogate mother, the Border collie Fly). But unlike the Gerber's commercials that feature mother and child ensconced in an immaculate nursery, cocooned together by the accoutrements of cozy furniture, perfectly tended plants, good hair and skin, *Babe*'s images of caring and intimacy do not work through sugarcoating but by keeping the darker realities always on the horizon. They are the reason we need to take care of one another.

*Babe* is, of course, a success story. But unlike *Rocky, Flashdance, Braveheart,* and the many other fantasies of empowerment in which socially underprivileged heroes and heroines rise above their circumstances and transform themselves through discipline, will, and dazzling physical prowess, *Babe* is a fable about the power of "difference," of nonassimilation. The polite little pig, who talks to the sheep rather than snaps and barks, turns out to be a better herder than the bossy Border collies! And in a significant way he transforms the culture and the values of the world he lives in. (It is suggested both at the beginning and the end of the film that attitudes toward pigs were never the same after *Babe* won the competition.) The *Rocky* model of success, like the "power feminism" model, is one of "making it" in a world that remains unchanged while the hero or heroine's body transforms itself to meet— and perhaps even surpass—the requirements of that world. This success is what we celebrate when female athletes demonstrate that they can develop the strength and power of men, when "special" Olympians cross the finish lines in their competitions, when those who have struggled to lose weight finally squeeze into those size-eight Calvin Kleins; the "outsider" is included by showing that he or she can "do it" too—on the terms of the culture. When the media celebrates such successes (and I do not deny that they are cause for celebration, as dramas of individual will, courage, and dedication), it usually leaves those cultural terms unquestioned.

*Babe* illustrates a different kind of success, one in which the "it" (of "Just Do It," "making it," "going for it") is interrogated and challenged. Those collies own the world (their own little world, that is) by virtue of their physical prowess and aggression, which—until *Babe* comes along—are the dominant values of that world. No one could have imagined that sheepherding could be done in any other way. How many of us have found ourselves struggling to prove our worth in a world that does not value us or our contributions? Often, the pressure to conform is overwhelming. *Babe*, unable to transform his waddly little body and unwilling to transform his empathic little soul into a mean, lean, fighting machine, represents the possibility of resisting that pressure—and transforming "the way things are." In a culture in which people are shamed for their "defects" and differences and seek safety in conformity, this tale may be a fantasy. But it is a precious one, one more worthy of our imaginations and ambitions—and our children's, surely—than "Just Do It!"

*Babe* is a fable and presents its message through the conventions of that genre, not through gritty realism. A glorious triumph is the reward for the "alternative" values that the little pig represents. Few of us experience such definitive or resounding validation of our efforts. But it is not necessary to win the big race in order to transform "the way things are." All of us, in myriad small ways, have the capacity to make some difference, because nothing that we do is a self-contained, disconnected, isolated event. Seemingly minor gestures of resistance to cultural norms can lay deep imprints on the lives of those around us. Unfortunately, gestures of capitulation do so as well. Consider the message sent by the mother who anxiously monitors her own weight and ships her daughter off to Jenny Craig at the first sign that her child's body is less than willowy, or the father who teases his wife (perhaps in front of their daughter) for being "out of shape." I don't mean to sound harsh; these responses may reflect personal insecurity, concern about the social acceptability of loved ones, panic over a child's future. But when we demonstrate seamless solidarity with our culture of images, we make its reign over the lives of those we love just a little bit stronger. And we unwittingly promote for them a life on the cultural treadmill.

I have learned a great deal about the extremes of that treadmill existence from my students' journals and from conversations with them in my office. Yes, my students know that as long as they keep up their daily hours at the gym, they can feel pumped up, look like Madonna, and burn enough calories so perhaps they will not have to throw up after dinner. But how, they wonder, can they possibly keep it up their entire lives? They know there is no equilibrium there, that the conditions of their feeling all right about themselves are *precarious*. It is here that *Babe* can speak to the situation of those who try to stop the breasts from sagging, thighs from spreading, wrinkles from forming. The parable not only makes visible more basic struggles that our obsession with appearance masks but also presents us with a metaphor for the *pathos* of that seemingly "superficial" obsession. The little pig performs in the final competition without any solid assurance of a happy ending. Even as he herds the sheep into the pen, he has not been told, in so many words, that he will be spared the carving knife. He wins the sheepherding trials, and, as is customary, the farmer utters the standard words "real" dogs hear at the end of their runs. "That'll do, Pig. That'll do." A formality usually—but in the context of *Babe*'s long struggle, these words say more, both to *Babe* and to the viewer. They represent, I believe, an acknowledgment that so many of us fervently long for in our lives—and are so rarely given. So many of us feel like *Babe*, trying our hardest to become something valued and loved, uncertain about whether we will ever be granted the right to simply exist. "That'll do. That'll do." These are words to break the heart. Enough. You've worked hard enough. I accept you. You can rest.

# NOTES

**1.** See Mareene Goodman, "Social, Psychological, and Developmental Factors in Women's Receptivity to Cosmetic Surgery," *Journal of Aging Studies* 8, no. 4 (1994): 375–96.

**2.** Quoted in Sally Ogle Davis, "Knifestyles of the Rich and Famous," *Marie Claire*, May 1996, p. 46.

**3.** Interview with Amanda de Cadenet, *Interview*, August 1995.

**4.** Rush Limbaugh, in his tirades against feminists and the academic left, has apparently not noticed that among these groups too the "victim" is not politically correct but passe. In the 1990s, postmodern academics look around and see not "oppressive" systems (which would be old-fashioned and "totalizing," so very "1960s") but "resistance," "subversion," and "creative negotiation" of the culture. (These academics may balk at being lined up on the side of *Braveheart* and Nike; they might also be surprised at how often the trope of cultural "resistance" appears in automobile ads.) In exalting the creative power and efficacy of the individual, the right and left—polarized around so many other issues—seem to be revelers at the same party.

**5.** Naomi Wolf, *Fire with Fire,* (New York: Random House, 1993), p. 45.

**6.** Debra Rosenberg et al., "Sexual Correctness," *Newsweek*, October 25, 1993, 56.

**7.** Kathy Davis, *Reshaping the Female Body: The Dilemma of Cosmetic Surgery* (New York: Routledge, 1995), 60–62.

**8.** See "Material Girl: The Effacements of Postmodern Culture," in my *Unbearable Weight* (Berkeley: University of California Press, 1993).

**9.** In 1994, there were nearly 400,000 aesthetic cosmetic surgeries performed in the United States, of which 65 percent were done on people with family incomes under $50,000 a year, even though health insurance does not cover cosmetic surgery. At the same time the number of people who say they approve aesthetic surgery has increased 50 percent in the last decade. See Charles Siebert, "The Cuts That Go Deeper," *New York Times Magazine*, July 7, 1996, pp. 20–26, 40–44.

**10.** Diana Dull and Candace West's research suggests that while "limited economic resources may *hinder* the pursuit of cosmetic surgery, they do not necessarily *prevent* that pursuit." They cite cases of people who have taken out loans for breast augmentations or who have scrimped and saved for years for their operations. See their "Accounting for Cosmetic Surgery: The Accomplishment of Gender," *Social Problems 18*, no. 1 (February 1991): 54–70.

**11.** In S. O. Davis, "Knifestyles," *Marie Claire*, May 1996, p. 46.

**12.** Amy Spindler, "It's a Face-Lifted, Tummy-Tucked Jungle Out There," *New York Times*, Sunday, June 9, 1996, pp. 6–10.

**13.** Quoted in Patricia Morrisroe, "Forever Young," *New York,* June 9, 1986, p. 47.

**14.** Letty Cottin Pogrebin, *Getting Over Getting Older,* (New York: Little Brown, 1996), 132.

**15.** Lily Burana, "Bend Me, Shape Me," *New York*, July 15, 1996, pp. 30–34.

**16.** Holly Brubach, "The Athletic Aesthetic," *New York Times Magazine*, June 23, 1996, pp. 48–51.

GERALD P. McKENNY

# Enhancements and the Ethical
# Significance of Vulnerability

It is an inescapable fact of life that our aims, desires, and projects all depend to one degree or another on the functioning of our bodies, and that our bodies are notoriously unreliable in enabling us to secure these aims, desires, and projects. At the limit, our bodies, whether by a native incapacity or by a sudden change, can bring to ruin our pursuit of highly valued activities or kinds of life. Consider the following scenarios: I return to the tennis court after several years and find that I am no longer quick enough to return the serves I once could. I begin study of a new language and find that my memory is not as capable of absorbing new vocabulary as some of my classmates. I am a crack reporter for a local news station but find that my face is unsuitable for a coveted position as an anchor. Cases like these remind us that our aims, desires, and projects are in effect hostages of our bodies. Our bodies, moreover, are themselves hostages of fortune: we are born with certain capacities and not others, and we have limited control over the incidence, and effects, of accident, aging, and disease. Yet even short of this limit, our bodies make it difficult to realize our aims and ideals even when they do not prevent us from realizing them. I may finally succeed at running a marathon or learning a foreign language, but only at an enormous expenditure of time and effort.

Various enhancement technologies now promise to reduce the obstacles our bodies present by optimizing certain performances (e.g., anabolic steroids), altering appearance (e.g., plastic surgery), or controlling features of one's personality (e.g., Prozac). These technologies fuel our confidence in the capacity of medicine to overcome what were once thought to be inherent limitations of our bodies. For some, the confidence brings with it an anxiety: even a thinker like Donna Haraway, who cautiously applauds what she heralds as the "cyborgian" erasure of the line between human and machine, worries that we might be in danger of denying our bodily vulnerability.[1] Yet, why should we be anxious about this prospect? If enhancements could guarantee, or (more likely) significantly improve the odds, that we will attain our aims and desires, and can remove or (more likely) significantly reduce the resistance our bodies present to our pursuit of these aims and desires, why should this not, other things being equal, be an unambiguous reason in their favor?

Most discussions of the ethics of enhancements focus on standard bioethical topics: questions regarding consent, risks and benefits, fairness in distribution, and so on. Meanwhile, it seems clear that a strong motivation for the use of enhancements is their efficacy (or perceived efficacy) in overcoming both the vulnerability of our bodies to fortune (which can prevent us from realizing our aims and ideals), and the resistance our bodies offer to our various pursuits (which makes it so difficult to realize our aims and ideals). Yet this motivation itself is almost never subjected to an ethical evaluation. Are the vulnerability and resistance of our bodies merely obstacles to be overcome to whatever extent possible? Or are vulnerability and resistance sources of self-regarding and other-regarding ethical values that are imperiled by attitudes and practices that view them only as obstacles to be overcome?

In this essay I want to explore the latter claim. It is important, however, to be clear about my target. My concern here is not what might happen should enhancements actually succeed in eliminating vulnerability and resistance. I believe, and at some crucial points the arguments I present presuppose, that they will not; that the body will always present an obstacle to the fulfillment of our aims and desires. Rather, my concern is with our attitudes and practices regarding the body and its place in an ethically worthy life: what role do its capacities and limitations play in an ethically worthy life, and how should our view of the ethical significance of our bodily capacities and limitations govern our use of the capacities of medicine, including enhancements? Included in this question is the possibility, denied or ignored by most moral evaluations of enhancements, that the limitations of our bodies (in this case, their vulnerability and resistance) with regard to our aims and desires might have ethical significance that is imperiled by efforts (whether successful or not) to overcome all such limitations. As I have indicated, it is this possibility that I wish to explore here.

In what follows I examine various philosophical positions that find ethical significance in the kind of vulnerability and resistance I have described. I begin with those views that concentrate on the resistance our bodies offer to the pursuit of our aims and ideals. I then turn to those views that focus on the vulnerability of our bodies to the fortune-governed factors that prevent us from attaining our aims and ideals. After this, I turn to the modern approach to fortune, to which I trace our attitudes and practices regarding enhancements. I close with a postmodern philosophical position that begins with a critique of a key element in the modern position. Three important qualifications must be indicated at the outset. First, I address only philosophical positions here, despite the fact that religious traditions have often had some of the most profound things to say about the issues I address. However, at least in the case of Christianity, they interact in very complex ways with several of the philosophical traditions treated here, so that it seemed more economical for a brief treatment of these issues to begin with the latter. Second, I offer nothing resembling a comprehensive treatment of the positions I survey. I am interested only in presenting the case I think each makes, or would make, for the ethical significance of vulnerability or resistance. Third, none of the positions I survey can be used in any direct way to determine specific judgments about particular kinds of enhancements or to arrive at a set of morally relevant distinctions that would enable one to classify kinds of enhancements. For some people, of course, this limitation is fatal. But the positions I treat here are only concerned with the attitudes, practices, dispositions, and beliefs that figure in our use of enhancements. If we get these right, the theory goes, we will be capable of making appropriate judgments about how to use enhancements and what role (if any) to assign them in our lives.

## The Resistant Body

A frequent reply to those who express reservations about modern technological forms of enhancement is that medicine has always been used for purposes of enhancement. To a certain extent it is true; premodern debates about the proper role of medicine in a morally worthy life often presupposed that adhering to a regimen could equip one for certain ways of life rather than others. In its attention to regimen, premodern medicine went beyond narrow concerns with restoring bodily functions when breakdowns occurred to concerns with cultivation of a body that would support valued activities or a specific way of life. Our contemporary preoccupation with enhancements, then, recalls those historical periods in which medicine—whether in cooperation or competition with philosophy and religion—was at the center of highly contested ethical debates about what kind of activities or way of life one should cultivate. So far, then, it appears that the chief difference between the ancients and ourselves is not the attention we give to enhancing the body but the fact that medicine, philosophy, and to a large extent even religion have, in our world, largely abandoned the task of articulating and debating views of the good life. Hence we and the ancients seem to be alike in our practice of enhancements, differing only in that we, unlike them, have no framework or discourse within which to judge which enhancements will contribute to a morally worthy life and which will detract from it.

However, a closer examination of premodern views indicates that the matter is not this simple. Three questions regarding the role of the body in a morally worthy life recur in premodern debates: Which of the capacities of medicine should we and should we not make use of? How much vigilance should we exercise over our bodies in accordance with the dictates of physicians? And finally, how should we respond to the susceptibility of our bodies to fortune? The first two questions were answered by placing the body in a teleological framework. For Plato, it was clear that the life of the guardians whose role he described in Book IV of the *Republic* required a different sort of medical training than that required for the life of the athlete. The preferred regimen of the athlete enhanced the performances of the body in ways Plato thought excessive and overly specialized. Likewise, it involved too much vigilance: those who followed it were required to devote too much attention to their bodies and too little to virtue. More than fifteen-hundred years later, Moses Maimonides made very similar arguments in reference to the kind of regimen appropriate to the life of the Jewish sage: a certain degree of bodily performance was necessary to pursue knowledge of God, but beyond this, the striving for higher levels of performance and the attention and esteem devoted to the body in order to attain these levels detracted from the proper goal.[2]

In principle, then, if we know the telos of our life, we should be able to judge, with greater or lesser degrees of specificity, the kinds of enhancements that would further our moral formation in light of that telos and the kinds that would detract from it. The response to these two questions by Plato and Maimonides therefore seems to confirm the view that the difference between them and us lies in our lack of such a teleological framework. But there are other differences as well, and at least some of these—the ones I underscore here—involve the body as an obstacle to our aims. The concern regarding excessive vigilance over or attention to the body reflects the sheer amount of time, effort, and devotion a regimen can demand. And this in turn results from the body's resistance to attempts to enhance it. Diet, exercise, control of sleep—these and other elements of classical regimen all require ongoing effort exerted against natural forces that constantly resist and reassert themselves against such effort. On the positive side of the ledger, this struggle against the body's natural resistance meant that adhering to such a regimen enabled one to cultivate the virtue of moderation or temperance, which was a strong argument in favor of regimen. On the negative side, the struggle could sap all the soul's energy and divert it from the higher concerns to which bodily well-being was generally subordinated—a strong reason for limiting one's regimen and assigning a lesser role to the improvement of the body and its capacities.

The need to struggle against the resistance of the body, then, set the agenda for ethical evaluations of traditional kinds of enhancement. By contrast, many of our enhancements are designed precisely to elimi-nate this need to struggle against a recalcitrant body. Their operation requires little or no ongoing effort on our part (though of course their ultimate effectiveness in terms of their contribution to the success of our projects may still require our effort). This, too, has its apparent advantages and disadvantages. On the negative side, we must worry about whether certain achievements—most obviously those involving athletic strength or capacity of memory—will continue to have the same meaning if the resistance of the body to those achievements is overcome by technological means that do not require our effort. On the positive side, the elimination of (at least some of) the need to struggle against the body holds out the promise that we need no longer devote so much ongoing attention to a recalcitrant body; time and effort can now be directed toward those things for which we value a high-performing body or toward enjoying one that conforms to our ideals. However, this optimistic result is not guaranteed: one can easily imagine us becoming obsessed with fine-tuning our bodies and, to that end, with refining and perfecting our enhancement technologies to the highest degree possible. This would in turn require continuous vigilance and extensive monitoring of our bodies and their performances.[3]

Beyond the comparison of these positive and negative features of each kind of technology of enhancement is a fundamental shift in the relation to the body in the pursuit of the good, and therefore in the view of the ethical significance of the body. The shift is this: Traditional techniques of enhancement required one to cultivate virtues such as moderation, so that the process by which one attained human fulfillment constituted an important part of that fulfillment itself. By contrast, to the extent that our technologies make it possible to enhance the self by acting directly on the body, they bypass the acting subject. And to that extent, human fulfillment—the realization of our aims and ideals— becomes a product rather than also a process, and the body a mere means rather than an integral component of self-formation.

## Vulnerability to Fortune

The third question, concerning a proper response to the susceptibility of the body to fortune, involved a different set of issues. Neither the given constitution of one's body nor the changes induced by disease, accident, and aging are fully, or even significantly, under one's control; fortune plays a major role in their distribution and effects. As such, fortune posed for premodern people the constant threat not only of resisting but of preventing altogether the attainment of one's aims and desires. To some extent, this question was also a teleological question: the inevitability of fortune is something one must consider in determining what bodily goods to pursue and how much vigilance to exercise. But the question of fortune also required a different kind of answer: one not only had to determine which ends are appropriate but to place the body in a hermeutical and practical framework in which its vulnerability to fortune could be understood and the anxiety it provoked overcome.

One such framework in the ancient world denies that things subject to fortune can possibly have any great significance for our lives. For the Stoics, eudaemonia, or happiness, is identical with the virtuous will and with the exercise of whatever degree of reason one is capable of.[4] These alone are intrinsically good, and they can be realized under almost any circumstances of life. Therefore, to treat bodily and external goods as if they were either intrinsically good (and thus comparable to virtue) or instrumentally good (that is, necessary for the attainment of virtue) is to act from false beliefs about their status as goods. One who treats such things as genuine goods subordinates oneself to what one does not directly control and becomes a slave of passions such as anger, grief, envy, and discontent, which are excited by the vicissitudes of fortune. The Stoic self was formed in part by rigorous practices of self-examination in which one distinguished between what depends on oneself and what does not, rejecting the latter as unworthy of one's desire or aversion.[5] The task is to attain self-mastery with regard to all that is external to virtuous reason, a self-mastery that is measured by one's lack of concern for all that is subject to fortune.[6]

None of this means that the Stoics had no use for medicine or that improving the body had no place in their scheme. Bodily and external goods such as health are not genuine goods, and are thus ultimately indifferent to our happiness, but they are to be preferred to their opposites. This notorious (and notoriously difficult) doctrine of the "preferred indifferents" is an enduring topic of scholarly debate. However one understands it, it seems clear that for the Stoics it is only when we have correct views about the goods of the body—that is, only when we recognize that such goods cannot secure or even contribute to our happiness—that we are in a position to make correct choices with regard to such goods and to help others to do the same. From this perspective, the Stoics might be in a position to criticize, on both self-regarding and other-regarding grounds, not so much enhancements themselves, but the attitudes that seem inseparable from our use of them. For in our pursuit of enhanced bodily performance and appearance, we may be trying to attain a kind of control over our lives that, according to the Stoics, is possible only through virtue. In enhancing our bodies, we seek to bring our bodies within the control of our will, so that they will be and do what we want them to be and do. But our bodies eventually betray us at some point: we may make temporary gains against natural necessity, but these gains only make us less prepared to face the vicissitudes of fortune when they come, as they inevitably will.[7] In pursuing enhancements in the false belief that what they secure really matters, we make it more likely that we will respond in anger when our bodies do fail us, envy when others appear or perform better than us, and discontent when enhancements do not do all that we want them to. And these passions, needless to say, harm not only ourselves but can lead to the harm of others as well.

What, then, is the proper Stoic attitude toward those who suffer from bodily conditions that prevent them from realizing their purposes in life? Insofar as these purposes accord genuine value to goods other than virtue itself, to relieve this kind of suffering can be destructive in two ways. First, it can perpetuate in the objects of our compassion the false notion that such things are of great importance, and by the same token prevent them from coming to realize what is truly important. Second, it can keep them dependent on things that are still beyond their control and thus inhibit their progress toward self-mastery. In short, enhancing any characteristic that is not constitutive of a virtuous soul may actually increase suffering. Instead, the proper relation to the other takes the form of bringing the other to acknowledge the futility of worrying about what is insignificant, leading ultimately to a more egalitarian friendship of self-commanding masters free from concern over fortune's whims.[8]

The Stoics developed their view in part in opposition to certain views of Aristotle and his followers, who represent a great rival solution to the problem of fortune.[9] It is clear that for Aristotle certain goods subject to fortune, such as friendship, are instrinsic components of happiness. The status of other such goods, such as bodily health, is less clear, but it is certain that they are at least instrumental to our happiness and, in some degree, necessary conditions of it. Some degree of bodily capacity, therefore, is necessary for happiness. However, the capacity needed is limited. Aristotle's view of happiness casts doubt on the contribution many of our aims and ideals make to our happiness. Since some degree of health, wealth, and beauty is instrumental, and even necessary, to our happiness, those who are severely deprived of these things may be inhibited in their capacity for happiness. But Aristotle was convinced that common opinion greatly overvalues these goods in a way that leads most of us to pursue them to the detriment of our happiness. On this reading, an Aristotelian might view enhancements as appropriate for the severely deprived (however we would have to determine who fits this description, and in what respects), but as unnecessary for the ethical well-being of the rest of us.

Not only would enhancements be unnecessary for those who are not severely deprived: an Aristotelian might also be deeply worried about what would happen if our use of enhancements led us to the belief (whether true or not) that our bodies were invulnerable to fortune. Martha Nussbaum points out that for Aristotelians, the socially necessary emotion of pity had three cognitive components: beliefs that the suffering of others for which pity is the appropriate response (1) is undeserved, (2) involves the loss of something valuable or important for one's life, and (3) is a kind of suffering that one recognizes could also happen to oneself.[10] The third belief is significant in this connection. If one is aware, in the midst of one's achievements, that one might not have achieved these things—that the necessary bodily conditions for one's achievements may have been lacking or taken away at fortune's whim—one is, on this theory, more likely to feel compassion for those who have been fortune's victims and have therefore not achieved as much. But what if we use enhancements in a way that leads us to deny the body's vulnerability to fortune? Having achieved what we have achieved largely without a sense that fortune could have or could still deprive us of our achievements, will we lose the chief source of our capacity to care for others, especially for lower achievers who (inevitably) will still be among us? The question is an empirical one, resting on a psychological thesis about the relation of a belief and an emotion, so it is unlikely we would know the answer. And, of course, the Stoics among us would question the value of this emotion anyway, inasmuch as it leads us to ascribe value to what fortune controls. But for non-Stoics, it is a question worth asking.

## Modernity and the Effort to Overcome Fortune

Once again, our debates over enhancements differ from those of the premodern world, for most of us deny that the subjection of our bodies to fortune has any positive role in directing us to our good, and this denial has important self-regarding and other-regarding implications just as the opposite affirmation does. In this connection it is important to remember how crucial it was for early modern thinkers such as Francis Bacon and Rene Descartes to redirect intellectual and practical endeavors to overcoming the subjection of life in general, and the body in particular, to fortune. Bacon and Descartes assign medicine a primary role in liberating humans from vulnerability to fortune, eventually leading to a culture in which, in Michel Foucault's terms, health replaces salvation: the vulnerability of the body to fortune is met as a condition to be eliminated by medicine rather than as an ineluctable feature of life to be addressed by moral or spiritual self-formation.[11] Moreover, for Descartes the way to overcome such vulnerability was to treat the body as an inanimate corpse, the object of a third-person gaze—an approach that reached its zenith in the work of Xavier Bichat a century and a half later. Implicit in this position is the reduction of the body to an object of control, making it plausible to conceive of medicine as a way of eliminating fortune and bringing the body under the power of our individual choices.

This modern view reveals a relation between one's attitudes and practices regarding bodily vulnerability and one's moral responsibilities regarding vulnerable others. Two immediate points are relevant here. First, the modern position assumes that the body is an important component, whether intrinsically or instrumentally, in the attainment of our aims. It follows that fortune can prevent us from attaining the good—a view, we have seen, that is not uncontested in Western thought. Compassion therefore takes the form of an imperative to eliminate fortune, as far as is possible and other things equal, from human life. Second, the discourses and techniques involved in capturing the body fully in the third person—the theoretical and practical rendering of the body as an object of control—are closely bound up with practices designed to optimize the capability of bodies. These practices trade on an irony in modern cultures: While our overt theories refrain from articulating a substantive view of the good within which bodily capacities and incapacities receive ethical significance, and claim instead to allow everyone to pursue their individual views of the good (and thus of the role of the body in that view), modern cultures carry out their own ambitions precisely by stimulating our desires, for ourselves and our offspring, for a certain kind of body, promoted through everything from advertising to health information campaigns. The result is that we express our concern for the bodily vulnerability of the other by seeking to ensure that his or her body measures up to norms designed to render our bodies maximally productive, useful, and efficient. This position is basically Foucault's analysis; I wish here only to highlight the other-regarding posture it implies: We respond to bodily vulnerability by measuring individuals against such norms and helping them to approximate them to the highest degree possible.

## Vulnerability and the Ethics of Alterity

There is a final feature of the modern effort to master fortune that leads to a very different kind of argument for the ethical significance of vulnerability. The modern commitment to overcoming fortune is part of a broader tendency to grant moral primacy to securing the conditions that preserve and enhance human life.[12] Many modern moral theories, including that of Thomas Hobbes, accordingly take as primary a (negative) right to that which preserves one's life, subject to limitations imposed by the presence of others who possess the same right. As is well known, the attention given to self-preservation expanded into a preoccupation also with self-expression, so that negative rights are increasingly extended to cover what one seeks for one's own individual self-fulfillment. In this context, the use of enhancements to overcome the subjection of our bodies to fortune can be seen as a way to secure more completely the conditions for self-preservation and self-expression, and the ethical evaluation of enhancements will begin with a presumption in their favor (whereas the Stoic and Aristotelian positions would most likely begin with some suspicion of them).

Emmanuel Levinas takes on this modern view that ethics begins with our (negative) entitlement to what fulfills our aims and purposes, subject only to the limitations posed by the similar entitlement of others.[13] For Levinas, this view defines human beings in terms of a *conatus essendi*, an interest in persisting in being. As such it marks the culmination of the Western philosophical tradition, which has always subordinated ethics to ontology or metaphysics with the result that the irreducible otherness of the human other has always been absorbed into the sameness of an order of being (in the form of a metaphysical order, the state, or an ideal of humanity, for example). In the face of the catastrophic results (ranging from colonialism to National Socialism) of the effort to assimilate otherness to the sameness of being, Levinas wants, like Kant, to affirm the priority of ethics to ontology. This move in turn requires an ethic that breaks with the primacy of the *conatus*. And it means going "beyond being" in order to establish the ethical relation as the transcendental ground of being.

To understand Levinas, and in particular to grasp the ethical signifi-cance of vulnerability in his thought, it may help to begin with the subordination of ethics to ontology. According to Levinas, Western philosophers from Plato and Aristotle through Descartes, Kant, Hegel, Husserl, and Heidegger have all offered one or another form of a philosophy grounded in ontology, in which the key move is to articulate the presence of being to consciousness or language. Being in these theories is dispersed through its appearances in time (think, for example, of the temporal character of our experience); and philosophy articulates the way in which consciousness or language recovers being from its dispersal by a unifying act of knowing or representation. As philosophers in the Continental tradition might put it, the presence of being, which is threatened by its diachronous dispersion, is secured by the synchronous capacity of a knowing consciousness or a representing language. (What is diachronous happens *over* or *through time*; what is synchronous happens *in* or *at the same time*.) The grounding of ethics in ontology occurs through the notion of the subject implied in this primacy of ontology. Correlative to this adventure of being is a subject who is formed by a similar resolution of diachrony into synchrony, which assures his place in the presence of being. Whether in the form of consciousness (through acts of retention or memory and protention or anticipation) or language (as a system of representation), the subject gathers itself up from the temporal dispersion of its experience into a unity in the presence of being. The diachrony of passing time (in which the past is irrevocably past and the future is always not yet, so that the subject can never coincide with itself) is recouped in consciousness and language that, to the extent they succeed, resolve the passing time of experience into the synchronous present of knowing and representation (in which the subject coincides with itself in the presence of being). In this way the subject secures itself by securing its persistence in being. The subject, then, is correlative to the presence of being, and is defined ontologically: the being of the subject is its persistence in being. The nature and task of ethics follows accordingly: ethics is grounded in the interest of the subject in persisting in being and takes the form of resolving conflicts between subjects who have a fundamental interest in persisting in being.

In contrast to this long Western philosophical tradition, Levinas shows that on reflection being is not really the first principle. Language, for example, signifies being only in the act of my signifying to another person; the latter is the condition of the possibility (the transcendental ground) of the former. Crucially, the latter—the signifying to the other—is not recouped in the former: the content that is signified depends on, but does not itself include, the act of signifying. Moreover, the act of saying is a passing over from myself to the other and is an exposure to the other: When I signify to the other I open myself up to and become vulnerable to the other. Saying is a nonrecriprocal being-for-the-other. Finally, the saying *qua* saying is not gathered up into what is said. The passivity of this passed time—the time elapsed in saying—is really time passed; diachrony is the ground of a synchrony that, contrary to the philosophical tradition, never does recoup it. Similarly with consciousness: the intentionality that grasps phenomena in terms of meanings depends upon the prior vulnerability of sensibility. Sensibility in the sense of being affected by something—feeling—is not recouped in meaning—in what is felt. The time passed in being affected is not recovered in what is felt; again, diachrony is the ground of a synchrony that never recoups it.

But if in these various ways diachrony is prior to and never recouped by synchrony, it follows that the ethical is prior to the ontological. For these various kinds of diachrony indicate that corporeality (e.g., sensibility, the passivity of passing time) is prior to language and con-sciousness, and this corporeality is ethical in character: the vulnerability of the body—its susceptibility to what affects it and to the passing of time—signifies, prior to the signification of a thing by sensible intuition, the one-for-the-other. The vulnerability of the body in sensibility is openness to the other. This other-regarding character of bodily vulnerability is abundantly clear here: "The body is neither an obstacle opposed to the soul, nor a tomb that imprisons it, but that by which the self is susceptibility itself. Incarnation is an extreme passivity; to be exposed to sickness, suffering, death, is to be exposed to compassion, and, as a self, to the gift that costs."[14] In short, the subject as openness to the other is prior to, and the condition of, the subject as consciousness and language, present to itself—the subject grounded in the *conatus*. That is an original nonreciprocal ethical relation, myself for another, is prior to, and the ground of, the reciprocity of selves persisting in being.

The vulnerability of the body thus has a privileged place in Levinas's philosophy, and from this place it challenges what he sees as the basic presuppositions of modern thought that have replaced the teleological orientation of ancient thought. According to these presuppositions, we are all fundamentally self-interested beings who seek to secure our place in a competitive world, and who therefore begin with a prima facie justification for enhancing our bodies in order to do so, so long as it does not threaten the fragile order that keeps conflicting interests from erupting into violence. But for Levinas, I begin not with my interest in securing my place in the world, but with my being for the other. From this perspective, my vulnerable body is the basis of my subjectivity. It does not call for remedy through enhancements that enable me to fulfill my interests. Nor does it call for narratives that make my suffering meaningful. Rather, it is precisely the fact that it is not overcome and not rendered meaningful that makes it possible for my suffering to be suffering for the other—even suffering for the suffering of the other—and thus an acceptance rather than a denial of my subjectivity. To seek to overcome this kind of vulnerability is to deny one's subjectivity and to submerge oneself and the other in the said and the felt, where being assigns its place to each of us.

However, this intractability is not the end of the story. Just as for Kant the fact of obligation is ultimately expressed in the universal, so for Levinas in actual life I am always for the other in the presence of the third person, who is also the other, and for whom I and the other are also other. At this level I must take account of multiple others, including myself as an other. At this level I must decide which instances of suffering deserve my priority. Does this mean that Levinas has simply given us an elaborate introduction to what in the end will be a classification of enhancements based on standard concerns regarding risks, benefits, and distribution? Not entirely. For the subject who prioritizes is never lost in the prioritization. Concretely, this means two things. First, for a subject constituted in this way, the default position is to live with one's vulnerability rather than to try to overcome it. Second, the nonreciprocality of this form of subjectivity means that one cannot expect this of others, only of oneself. The burden of proof is therefore on those who would deny the recourse of others to enhancements.

## Conclusion

I have tried in this essay to describe various perspectives on the vulnerability of the body from which that vulnerability has both self-regarding and other-regarding ethical significance. Among the three perspectives that find ethical significance in such vulnerability, there are crucial differences. For the Stoics, the ethical significance follows from the logic of their overall position, while for Aristotle it follows from a psychological thesis, and for Levinas it is a transcendental claim. None of the three positions rules out enhancements categorically or supports a clear classification or prioritization. Nevertheless, there is an important thread of continuity that deserves more attention in ethical debates over enhancements than it has received. The thread of continuity is the conviction that how we interpret and act upon our bodies has enormous significance for our moral identity. Consequently, the use we make of medicine is not merely a source of moral dilemmas that are dealt with on other grounds but is itself an important part of our moral formation. To the extent that enhancements overcome, or lead us to deny, the vulnerability of the body, they also foreclose the kinds of self-formation that our awareness of vulnerability makes possible. Prior to questions of how to classify and prioritize enhancements is the question of what kind of self we should cultivate through medicine.[15]

## Acknowledgment

The author thanks B. Andrew Lustig, Erik Parens, and members of The Hastings Center's "Enhancement Project" for their comments on earlier drafts of this essay.

## NOTES

**1.** Donna Haraway, *Simians, Cyborgs, and Women*, (New York: Routledge, 1991).

**2.** Moses Maimonides, *Ethical Writings of Maimonides*, edited by Raymond L. Weiss with Charles Butterworth (New York: Dover, 1975).

**3.** Of course, the extensive vigilance and monitoring is problematic only if the body is not itself the primary or ultimate end sought in enhancing it. The ancient view I am describing assumes that virtue is the primary or ultimate end, though this assumption need not preclude the body from being a genuine though subordinate part of the end.

**4.** The following portrait of Stoicism is something of a composite portrait. It is largely based on my reading of Seneca and Marcus Aurelius, and on the scholarship of Julia Annas, *The Morality of Happiness* (New York: Oxford University Press, 1993); Terrence Irwin, "Stoic and Aristotelian Conceptions of Happiness," in *The Norms of Nature* (New York: Cambridge University Press, 1986); and Martha Nussbaum, *The Therapy of Desire* (Princeton, N.J.: Princeton University Press, 1994).

**5.** Practices of this kind regarding the body can be found in the letters of Seneca and in Marcus Aurelius's Meditations.

**6.** The Stoic response to the vulnerability of the body is echoed in Nietzsche's well-known response to his incurable pain. Noting how his pain is loyal, obstrusive, shameless, yet also clever and entertaining, Nietzsche announces, "I have given a name to my pain, and call it 'dog,' " thereby asserting mastery—both in form and in content—over what he did not control. Quoted in David B. Morris, *The Culture of Pain* (Berkeley: University of California Press, 1991), p. 284.

**7.** In *The Culture of Pain*, David Morris points out that our quest to conquer pain has coincided with a dramatic increase, numerically and in magnitude, in pain-related problems, an increase Morris attributes in part to the expectation that pain could be eliminated.

**8.** The concern for the other is therefore concern for the other's effort to gain self-mastery over the vulnerability of the body. This concern for the other is apparent, again, in the letters of Seneca and perhaps, in a very different form, in the figure of Nietzsche's Zarathustra.

**9.** My presentation of the Aristotelian position is indebted to Julia Annas, *The Morality of Happiness*; Terrence Irwin, "Stoic and Aristotelian Conceptions of Happiness"; Martha Nussbaum, *The Fragility of Goodness* (New York: Cambridge University Press, 1986); and Martha Nussbaum, *The Therapy of Desire*.

**10.** Martha Nussbaum, *The Therapy of Desire*, p. 87.

**11.** Michel Foucault, *Birth of the Clinic* (New York: Random House, 1973).

**12.** Charles Taylor, in *Sources of the Self* (Cambridge: Harvard University Press, 1989) helpfully discusses this position under the heading of the moral significance of the pursuits of "ordinary life," which begins with the Protestant critique of the monastic ideal in favor of family life and work in a calling, and which continues through various forms of Enlightenment naturalism to the present.

13. My presentation of Levinas draws primarily from his *Totality and Infinity* (Pittsburgh: Duquesne University Press, 1969) and *Otherwise than Being, or beyond Essence* (The Hague: Martinus Nijhoff, 1981).

14. Levinas, *Otherwise than Being, or beyond Essence*, p. 195 n. 12.

15. I have argued this thesis in regard to medicine more generally in my book, *To Relieve the Human Condition* (Albany, N.Y.: State University of New York Press, 1997).

MARY G. WINKLER

# Devices and Desires
# of Our Own Hearts

*Tis all in pieces, all Coherence gone*
*All just supply, and all Relation.*

Reflections on enhancement technologies have a longer history than we often recognize. John Donne wrote *Anatomie of the World* in 1611 as part of a lament for a young girl. But he extends his meditations to the political and intellectual upheavals of his time, and he couches them in the metaphors of the new medical science: anatomy. As is well known, the lost coherence is the coherence of a cosmology that had long been understood to dictate terrestrial order. Donne and his contemporaries (at least those learned and/or leisured enough to be aware of astronomy) were still staggering from the blows to their understanding of the universe. No longer could they imagine themselves inhabitants of a static orb, at the center of a series of majestically wheeling concentric crystalline spheres. No longer could they look into the night sky and feel secure in the finitude of the cosmos. Now they must perceive a boundless, seemingly unending sea of space. No longer would they seek comfort in analogies between macrocosm and microcosm, in the understanding that each man is a little universe. The perceptual consequences, as Donne suggests, caused a sense of dislocation and dis-ease. In *The Discarded Image*, C.S. Lewis aptly draws the distinction between medieval and modern corporeal experience of the heavens:

> Hence to look out on the night sky with modern eyes is like looking over a sea that fades away into mist, or looking about one in a trackless forest—trees forever and no horizon. To look up at the towering medieval universe is much more like looking at a great building. The "space" of modern astronomy may arouse terror, or bewilderment or vague reverie;

the spheres of the old present us with an object in which the mind can rest, overwhelming in its greatness but satisfying in its harmony.[1]

The "'space' of modern astronomy" is (as we are well aware) a space made visible by technology. In 1610, when Galileo published *Siderius Nuncius*, the earliest published report of telescopic observations of the heavens, he began the process by which the old cosmology lost its validity as science. "O telescope," wrote Kepler, "instrument of much knowledge, more precious than any sceptre! Is not he who holds thee in his hand made king and lord of the works of God!"[2]

The terms of the debate were set early: Donne's lament and Kepler's encomium discover the poles between anxiety and confidence. Contemporary response to technology still explores the territory between them. In 1990, Sir Ian Lloyd echoed Donne in his speech before the House of Commons.

> As science takes us nearer to the fundamentals of creation, whether through the outward reach of the Hubble telescope . . . , or the inward reach of the scanning tunnel microscope, revealing for the first time the secrets of the living cell, we shall be presented with greater potential for good and evil, greater powers of intervention, and greater challenges to orthodox dogmas of all kinds—religious, scientific and political.[3]

A recent letter to the editor of *The New York Times* (March 9, 1997) responded to President Clinton's desire to prohibit federal research funding for human cloning. The author raises the specter of the Inquisition, accusing the President of "acting like a medieval theologian." He invites the reader to imagine "living at the time of Galileo's breakthrough and having government respond by banning the telescope!"[4]

No doubt many see the issue of enhancement technologies as a contest between the proponents of scientific progress and the advocates of tradition, cautious perspicuity or even superstition. But, of course, it is nowhere near that simple. Reflection on the telescope's development reveals subtleties that may be quite apropos to a discussion of contemporary enhancement technologies. The telescope—that previous "instrument of much knowledge"—began its history in a rather more humble service. The knowledge of lens grinding developed in response to a common and simple desire—the desire to slow the effects of presbyopia—elderly eyesight. At least three centuries before the telescope (as readers of *The Name of the Rose* remember), some elderly men wore magnifying eyeglasses. With these spectacles, scholars who once were forced into retirement by dimness of vision could remain at their desks.

The aged could continue participating, could read and study.[5] From this relatively simple technology for enhancing eyesight developed the telescope and the overthrow of an ancient cosmology. From this technology came also the microscope and scientific medicine rooted in the observation of the invisible. We at the end of the twentieth century no longer rhapsodize over the telescope—or the microscope for that matter. We have domesticated their powers and live our daily lives almost heedless of the ways they have altered not only our existence but our perceptions of ourselves. Yet, because of the telescope, we know ourselves to be infinitesimal beings in an unimaginably vast universe. We cannot, as ancient and medieval peoples could, innocently imagine humanity and human concerns to be central to the operation of the cosmos. Because of the microscope, our selves—our bodies—have become universes for exploration—our most minute and intimate reaches visible. We have been "anatomized" to a degree that John Donne could not envision even in his dreams.

John Donne was not wrong to perceive a loss—both to his contemporaries' sense of certainty and to their understanding of the self in society.

> For every man alone thinkes he hath got
> To be a Phoenix, and that there can bee
> None of that kinde, of which he is, but hee.

The medieval lens makers could no more imagine the consequences of their work than can those who create today's technologies and procedures. In the beginning, they worked in response to a simple human desire: let me not lose my eyesight with age. Let me retain the eyes of youth.

I introduce desire here because it is important to explore the desires that drive the invention or creation of new technologies. We create our devices in response to our desires. It is not enough to make divisions between progress and caution, to either promote or ban. Rather, it is useful to ask what need the new technologies fill. What impels the cultural demand for cosmetic surgery, for Prozac and other enhancing drugs, for genetic engineering? What desires do these demands reveal?

One place where our society finds its desires defined and reflected is advertising. Jean-Marie Dru, chairman of the French advertising agency B.D.D.P., makes the point succinctly: "Nothing reflects a country and an age better than its advertising."[6] In *Ways of Seeing*, the writer and critic John Berger makes pointed observations about advertising (or "publicity") and the buyer's desires.[7] Advertising seems, he writes, to offer choices and choices described in the language of freedom. But let the buyer beware. Beneath the seeming plethora of options is only a single proposal: the proposal that "we transform ourselves, or our lives, by buying something more." In order to pique desire for the transformation, advertising offers an image of an ideal self—a self perfected and liberated from the anxiety of imperfection. "Publicity [advertising] is never a celebration of pleasure-in-itself. It offers [the potential buyer] an image of himself made glamorous by the product or opportunity it is trying to sell. The image then makes him envious of himself as he might be."[8] Further: "The spectator-buyer is meant to envy herself as she will become if she buys the product. . . . One could put it another way: the publicity image steals her love of herself as she is, and offers it back to her for the price of the product."[9] And we should not forget that the products of technology are products—commodities.

Taking Berger's observations as a guide, one may ask what themes are to be found in advertising that speak to the desire for enhancement technologies? What transformations are desired? What opportunities are offered?

Even a superficial search in magazines and journals reveals one theme that recurs again and again in a surprisingly wide range of contexts. The theme is that of control. Everywhere purveyors of products promise the buyer control over everything from unruly hair to life-threatening illness. So prevalent is the concern with control, that it may be read as a topos of *fin de siecle* American culture.[10] And the locus of concern is the body—the individual is exhorted to turn to bodily control and enhancement as a response to social or political problems.

Anyone acquainted with the language of medical science is accustomed to the language of control. Thus it should not surprise us that advertisements for pharmaceutical products speak in that mode. The text of an advertisement for hypertension tablets is typical of many found in medical journals: "Sular for hypertension tablets. Control the course of therapy on your terms." ("The clinical profile you demand. A price today's changing environment requires.") Typical also is the language of an advertisement for asthma treatment: "Controlling asthma can be an uphill battle. The strength of Aerobid can make it easier. Aerobid—the strength to control asthma. With fewer puffs per day." Larger than the text and strong enough to carry the message is the photograph of a solitary young man vigorously running up a bank of

242 Mary G. Winkler

stadium steps. The image makes clear that he is midway in his course: many steps lie below him, many steps rise ahead. The image makes literal the metaphor "uphill battle" and thereby offers the asthma sufferer not merely control but conquest.

Pharmaceutical companies are not the only ones that promise solace of control. Dreyfus, a brokerage house, makes investors in the Lion Account this promise: "Introducing a single account that gives you the guidance and tools to control all your finances. Start to plan your future. . . . [T]he Lion Account offers you the tools to reach your goals and the power to control all your finances."

An advertisement for hair gel makes the concerns of the buyer even more explicit. "You never had this much control when you were on your own," triumphs the L'Oreal copy. "Mega Gel from Studio Line has plenty of control to go around. A source of strength. A source of power. So you can do things you never could before. It's a power trip all right. And everyone should take one. Because while we all could use control, some could use more than others."

The smoothly coiffed woman using Mega Gel has a male counterpart speaking on behalf of a Houston cosmetic surgeon. This handsome young professional looks into the camera and explains, "I'm a take-charge-kind-of-person. In every aspect of my life." Therefore, he has "made a few small changes that have made all the difference." "When you're on top of the world, you want an appearance that reflects your potential."

Looking beneath the surface for the locus of desire, one sees that all of the advertisements offer the buyer hope that he or she may have power over uncertainty or contingency. The individual desires may vary. One may hope for relief from a containment of a chronic disease. Another may wish for beautifully styled hair. Yet another may want the opportunity to advance in a career. Many may wish to avoid the ill consequences of a fluctuating economy.

Yet at their most fundamental, all of these advertisements address anxieties about adversity. "The way we see it, you face enough adversity in this world. You might as well be comfortable." This is an offer to the prospective owner of a Mercury Mountaineer: "When the going gets tough, the tough get comfortable." Here the copy co-opts medicine's language: "We cannot cure you, but we can make you comfortable." No doubt the advertisements trivialize our desires. But they also reveal their deeper significance. What are these desires, the fulfillment of which would make us envious of ourselves as we might be? Looking beneath the surface, beneath the desires for beauty, success, comfort, one can begin to perceive the deeper meaning of these ubiquitous offers of control. "Power over time," promises Lancome, "double performance, anti-wrinkle and firming treatment." With "age-defiant elements."

Power over time. Comfort in adversity. Autonomy. Escape from anxious care and concern. Protection against uncertainty. Love. These are the desires revealed in the mirror of the advertiser's copy. But there is more: the language is not the passive language of freedom. It is the active, restless language of conquest. One must control oneself, one's fate. One must buy something, *do* something. Here is where the culture of advertising and the desire for enhancement technologies begin their conversation. For like the hair gels and face creams, the automobiles and investment plans, the new technologies also appeal to the desire for control—and offer to allay our deepest fears.

It is useful to reflect on the history of the optical lens as exemplary of the paradoxical nature of enhancement technologies of all kinds. Discussants of new technologies often feel compelled to situate themselves somewhere on a continuum between desire and fear. One desires the benefits of new technology. One desires, for example, to have one's eyesight enhanced—to see beyond the capacity of the unaided human eye, to read the heavens, to know the infinitesimal. Such knowledge can be frightening, can overthrow entire intellectual systems, can make one giddy with a vision of chaos. Such knowledge can also liberate and heal.

It is never so simple as ranking the forces of superstition against the armies of science; of drawing a line between love of knowledge and hubris. Technologies are invented and employed in cultural contexts. And the cultural context of late twentieth-century American technological development is one in which desire for control struggles with an anxiety approaching terror. In the collage of popular culture one sees pieced together not only the fantasies of control but the agitated contemplations of disaster. Reviewing only the past year, one can find movie and television schedules filled with meditations on destruction—communities engulfed in molten lava (*Dante's Peak* and *Volcano*), destruction by asteroids (*Asteroid*), invasions of unappeasable alien forces (*Independence Day*), tornadoes and tidal waves. CBS recently (March 23, 1997) announced a news magazine discussion of the terrorist attack at the Empire State Building with this question: "Is any place safe from this kind of terror?" Man, Nature, and the cosmos run amok, uncontrollable.

"The sleep of reason produces nightmares," is the caption in one of Goya's dark *capriccios*. And, indeed, the unbounded longing for control has its twin specter of helplessness and disorder. If one can only anxiously shuttle between the poles of control and chaos, then one may well long for a stable resting place and for a refreshing sleep guarded by reason.

The name of *Brave New World* has been invoked so frequently since the cloning of the sheep and monkey, that I introduce it with caution. I introduce it, however, to investigate one of the themes of the novel. In chapter 16 a conversation takes place among Mustapha Mond, the Resident Controller for Western Europe (one of the ten world controllers), Helmholtz Watson, a lecturer at the College of Emotional Engineering and writer of radio programs, "feely" scenarios, slogans, and hypnopedic rhymes, and John, the Savage.[11] John, born after his mother, Linda, was left behind on the Malpais Reservation, has grown up a stranger both to the worlds of his mother and of the Indians among whom he lives. He has had neither the scientific conditioning of the England over which Mustapha Mond presides nor the traditional, part mystical teachings of the Pueblo culture. What he has had is Shakespeare, a somewhat mouse-nibbled volume, a relic of pre-brave-new-world civilization. In the interview, the Savage has just acknowledged that he does not like civilization, in spite of "some very nice things" such as the music in the air. The Controller responds by reciting Caliban's speech, "Sometimes a thousand twangling instruments will hum about my ears and sometimes voices." The Savage, joyfully imagining that he has at last found a kindred spirit, asks if the Controller has read "the book," too. Indeed he has—the Controller replies—he is one of the few people in England to whom the book is not forbidden.

The Savage is astounded. Why should such a book be prohibited? Because, says the Controller, it's old. Old things are of no use in his society. "Even when they are beautiful?" asks the Savage. "Particularly when they are beautiful." The Controller patiently explains. Contemplation of the beauty of old things will distract the people from the new. But the new things are "so stupid and horrible." Why not let the people see *Othello* instead? Again the Controller is patient. "I've told you; it's old. Besides, they couldn't understand it."

Undaunted, the Savage offers another option: Let writers write something *new* that is like *Othello*, but understandable. This animates Helmholz Watson and he joins the questioning "Why not?" "Yes, why not?" "Why not?"

The Controller's reply leads the reader into the heart of *Brave New World*.

> Because our world is not the same as Othello's world. You can't make flivvers without steel—and you can't make tragedies without social instability. The world's stable now. People are happy; they get what they want, and they never want what they can't get. They're well off; they're safe; they're never ill; they're not afraid of death; they're blissfully ignorant of passion and old age; they're plagued with no mothers or fathers; they've got no wives and children, or lovers to feel strongly about; they're so conditioned that they practically can't help behaving as they ought to behave.

The Savage reflects on this, and counters the Controller's sermon: "All the same, *Othello's* good, *Othello's* better than those feelies."

Indeed, agrees the Controller. But the renunciation of art—of tragedy—is the price we pay for stability. The work of Helmholtz Watson, for example, requires "the most enormous ingenuity." The writer in "civilization" must "make art out of nothing but pure sensation." The Savage remains unconvinced. What the Controller has described is "quite horrible."

The Controller acknowledges the Savage's response. Of course, happiness looks "pretty squalid" in comparison with "the over-compensations for misery." Contentment has "none of the glamour of a good fight with misfortune, none of the picturesqueness of a struggle with temptation, or a fatal overthrow by passion or doubt."

In *Brave New World* all things that hint at a fuller life are suppressed or hidden. Einstein and Picasso are as unwelcome as Shakespeare or, for that matter, John Donne. Consequently, there is no art, no religion, no true science. There is no love.

The advertisements for the control of unruly hair and unruly finances would be at home in Mustapha Mond's world were it not that the battle for control has already been fought and won there. In *Brave New World* people have the bodies society requires of them, and presumably the market does not fluctuate. But occasionally in their communal sleep Huxley allows even the happiest of individuals to experience an intimation of the fullness of the human condition. Lenina Crowne, the beautiful self-satisfied "pneumatic" Alpha is returning from an evening with Bernard Marx in Bernard's helicopter. Suddenly, Bernard has stopped his propeller, causing them to hover a hundred feet from the roiling English Channel. It is a cloudy night and the wind has risen.

Lenina's reaction is startling. "It's horrible," she repeats again and again, using the same words the Savage will find to describe the "art" of the Controller's civilization. "She was," writes Huxley, "appalled by the rushing emptiness of the night, by the black foam-flecked water heaving beneath them, by the pale face of the moon, so haggard and distracted among the hastening clouds. 'Let's turn on the radio, quick!' "[12]

When the title of Huxley's novel is invoked in the media, the invocation usually occurs in a story of some new morally ambiguous technology. Often, it is a facile invocation.

But a deeper reading indicates that the novel is Aldous Huxley's contemplation of a great and ancient question: What is the good life? Through satire, *Brave New World* explores a society that prizes stability above contingency, happiness above goodness. That is the burden of the dialogue between the Savage, John, and the Controller. The world the Controller describes is unbalanced. To achieve stability and control, the makers of the brave new world have lopped off all the parts of the human condition that allow ambiguity or transcendence.

Yet even there one finds a world beyond the closely circumscribed and controlled world over which Mustapha Mond presides. Lenina Crowne's horror at the night-dark stormy waves makes this clear. Her conditioning is perfect. She knows where to turn for solace—the technology is ready to hand. "Skies are always blue inside of you" warbles the radio singer. But she has had a moment of terror—a glimpse of a nature that is aeons old, and uncontrolled by the modes and laws of civilization. She has thereby had a moment of knowledge of herself as a person with emotions as dark and mysterious as the heaving channel itself.

When the nightly television newscaster invokes the name *Brave New World* to trigger audience response to the latest story of scientific or technological discovery, he is probably not expecting his audience to even have read *Brave New World*. The phrase has entered our cultural vocabulary. Everyone is expected to understand the shorthand. *Brave New World* means science run wild, social control through technology— babies in bottles, mad scientists playing God. But, of course, no one is expected to look within to see where his or her own desire for a brave new world might lie.

An advertisement for the services of another Houston cosmetic surgeon shows a bright-eyed, smiling young woman. She faces the camera confidently, but her arms are crossed at her waist. The text of the advertisement reads, "Beware the Thighs of March! Make a small change on the outside that could lead to BIG changes on the inside!" The thighs of the young woman are not visible in the photograph. That would distract from the invitation that the cosmetic surgeon offers. It is not really about thighs, or breasts, or tummies to be tucked, whispers the image. It is about an unburdened, confident self. The image of the frontally posed, smiling woman does not, however, welcome the approach of others. The nature of her confidence is expressed through her folded arms. It is a confidence won by surgical defense against imperfection. The BIG change inside is not achieved through a rigorous journey toward self-knowledge, nor through a politically engaged exploration of the reasons why a "better" body should make her more of a "success." One imagines that she has a lifestyle, not a life; and that the "could be" self the ad encourages her to envy is a person who need never experience a night sky or stormy sea within herself.

I am aware that I am about to launch into troubled waters myself as I conclude my reflections on control and technology. No discussion of the uses of enhancement technologies should ignore the very real suffering of individuals in late twentieth-century American society. I am very much in sympathy with Freeman Dyson's dictum. "As a general rule to which there are many exceptions, science works for evil when its effect is to provide toys for the rich, and it works for good when its effect is to provide necessities for the poor."[13] Yet, I would not ignore the desires of any—they are all human desires. And I remember that enhancement technologies like our simple eyeglasses appear in the uncharted border lands where desire and necessity meet. This fact the entrepreneur and the advertiser understand as well as the scientist, or the theologian.

The advertiser understands the fears and desires very well. In imagination I see a *Justitia*-like figure—the personification of advertising. She holds a scale in which societal anxieties are weighed against the products that will soothe them. Against fear of failure, aging and death, are weighed the creams, lotions, automobiles and—yes—medications, surgeries, and technologies that promise to allay fear and wipe the tears from our eyes.

In *Brave New World*, there are only two possibilities offered the human race: "World control and destruction."[14] The choice, of course, is control—control achieved with a vengeance. People are manufactured, conditioned to fit their proper societal niche, to know and desire nothing other. Liberty is only "liberty to be inefficient and miserable. Freedom to be a round peg in a square hole."[15] Aging is forbidden and death is hidden. Nothing messy or complex is allowed.

Huxley's novel is now sixty-five years old. Perhaps some of his vision seems outdated or extreme (his vision has its own historical context), but at the core of the novel we encounter the desires and fears familiar to our decade. Mustapha Mond promises the removal of all insurmountable obstacles, the collapsing of time between desire and fulfillment.[16] He promises the assuagement of "the primal and the ultimate need. Stability."[17] *Brave New World* is a world where technology reigns, but where full humanity is sacrificed to stability. Like the stability created by the balanced scales of my imaginal goddess of advertising, *Brave New World*'s stability offers no other good option.

But other options are available. Lenina Crowne's response to the stormy sea opens the door to reflection on one such option. She cannot experience nature except through sentimentality or with terror. Everything in her controlled society overtly conspires to prevent her having a full knowledge of the night. She turns to the saccharine music that soothes but forestalls direct experience of the natural world's power and grandeur. She does not, because she cannot, turn to Beethoven's Pastorale Symphony—to music that dares the heart of the storm, knows it, embraces its danger, borrows its exhilarating force, and finally comes to rest with the calm.

Do we think that by controlling the body we can control the heart? Perhaps that is the desire. But too often the manifestation of that desire is what Kathleen Norris has called "the bizarre idolatry of body parts."[18]

We cannot—and should not—put the genie back in the bottle. The genie is, after all, a servant. It is the master that sets the tasks. Therefore, if we want to use our technologies for good—not as toys or pacifiers, but as true enhancers of our brief lives—I suggest that we reflect on our "bizarre idolatries." The idolized body parts may be visible—breasts, thighs, height. Or they may be visible only through the microscope. The parts may be diseased, or merely lacking socially constructed "perfection." Contemplating them in isolation should give us pause: a human being is not merely the sum of her parts. Contemplating the human body only as an issue, a burden, or a problem to be solved often leads us in the direction of desire for control. Contemporary society is often in danger of idolizing not only body parts, but control itself.

This essay began with John Donne's lament for a dead girl and a lost world. His lament encompasses a personal grief and a revolution in understanding. We can alter the world with our loves and our desires. Simple magnifying lenses become the Hubble telescope and the most sophisticated microscopy. Donne was right to see the change: both outer and inner universes are more complex and mysterious than he or his ancestors imagined. In thinking about enhancement technologies, let us begin by acknowledging the mysteries of human existence. If we want to use our technologies well, let us not use them as retreats from societal complexity or as salves for the envy of impossibly ideal selves. If we want to use our technologies well, let us, rather, look at each technology and at each of its particular uses with these questions in mind: does the technology enhance the whole person, or does it offer only a palliative substitute for wholeness? Does it serve our desires for completeness and connection, or does it pander to our anxieties and our short-sighted demands for control? Finally, does the technology and its application help us to love and honor the body in all its fragility, imperfection, and finitude?

## NOTES

1. C.S. Lewis, *The Discarded Image: An Introduction to Medieval Renaissance Literature* (Cambridge: Cambridge University Press, 1964), p. 19.

2. Quoted in Allen G. Debus, *Man and Nature in the Renaissance* (Cambridge: Cambridge University Press, 1964), p. 96.

3. Sir Ian Lloyd, *Parliamentary Debates*, Commons, 6th Ser., Vol. 171 (1990) col. 96, quoted in Susan Merrill Squier, *Babies in Bottles: Twentieth-Century Visions of Reproductive Technology* (New Brunswick, N.J.: Rutgers University Press, 1994), p. 133.

4. Dennis G. Kuby, *The New York Times*, Editorials, March 9, 1997, p. 14.

5. Albert Van Helden, *The Invention of the Telescope: Transactions of the American Philosophical Society*, Vol. 67, Part 4 (1977), p. 10.

6. Quoted in John Heilemann, "Annals of Advertising: All Europeans Are Not Alike," *The New Yorker,* April 28 and May 5, 1997, p. 181. In the same article. Florence Waterman, European account director for McDonald's, is described as frequently citing Derrida and Foucault!

7. John Berger, *Ways of Seeing* (London: Penguin Books, 1982), p. 131.

8. Berger, *Ways of Seeing*, p. 132.

9. Berger, *Ways of Seeing*, p. 134.

10. The word "control" has an interesting etymology and history. It derives from the Latin "rotulus" (scroll) and makes its first appearance in the fourteenth century, according to the *Oxford English Dictionary*. By the late fifteenth century it has entered the vocabulary of bookkeeping and accounting. During the sixteenth century (i.e., the beginning of the rise of the bureaucratic state), the word begins to gain its modern connotations.

11. Aldous Huxley, *Brave New World and Brave New World Revisited* (New York: Harper Collins, 1965), pp. 168–70. All quotes are from this edition.

12. Huxley, *Brave New World*, p. 69.

13. Freeman Dyson, "Can Science Be Ethical?" *The New York Review of Books*, April 10, 1997, p. 47.

14. Huxley, *Brave New World*, p. 36.

15. Huxley, *Brave New World*, p. 34.

16. Huxley, *Brave New World*, p. 33.

17. Huxley, *Brave New World*, p. 31.

18. Kathleen Norris, *Cloister Walk* (New York: Riverhead Press, 1996), p. 325.

# Contributors

**Susan Bordo** holds the Otis A. Singletary Chair in the Humanities and is a professor of philosophy at the University of Kentucky, Lexington, Kentucky.

**Dan W. Brock** is director for the Center for Biomedical Ethics, a professor of philosophy and biomedical ethics, and a Charles C. Tillinghast, Jr., University Professor at Brown University, Providence, Rhode Island.

**Ronald Cole-Turner** is the H. Parker Sharp Associate Professor of Theology and Ethics at Pittsburgh Theological Seminary, Pittsburgh, Pennsylvania.

**Kathy Davis** is a professor on the Faculty of Social Sciences for Women's Studies Social Sciences at the University of Utrecht, Utrecht, the Netherlands.

**Carl Elliott** is a professor of philosophy and pediatrics at the Center for Bioethics at the University of Minnesota, Minneapolis, Minnesota.

**David M. Frankford** is a professor of law at Rutgers University School of Law-Camden, and a member of the graduate department of public policy and administration at the Institute for Health, Health Care Policy and Aging Research at Rutgers University, Camden, New Jersey.

**Carol Freedman** is an assistant professor of philosophy at Williams College in Williamstown, Massachusetts.

**Eric T. Juengst** is an associate professor of biomedical ethics at the Center for Biomedical Ethics, School of Medicine, Case Western Reserve University, Cleveland, Ohio.

**Margaret Olivia Little** is a senior research scholar at the Kennedy Institute of Ethics and an assistant professor in the Department of Philosophy at Georgetown University, Washington, D.C.

**Gerald P. McKenny** is an associate professor of religious studies at Rice University, Houston, Texas.

**Erik Parens** is associate for philosophical studies at The Hastings Center, Garrison, New York.

**Anita Silvers** is a professor of philosophy at San Francisco State University, San Francisco, California.

**Mary G. Winkler** is an associate professor at the Institute for the Medical Humanities, University of Texas Medical Branch, Galveston, Texas.

# Index